Concussion. Brain on Pause. How to Hit Play.

A Practical and Illustrated Guide to Overcoming Concussion, Post Concussion Syndrome (PCS), and Mild Traumatic Brain Injury (mTBI).

Paul Godlewski, PT

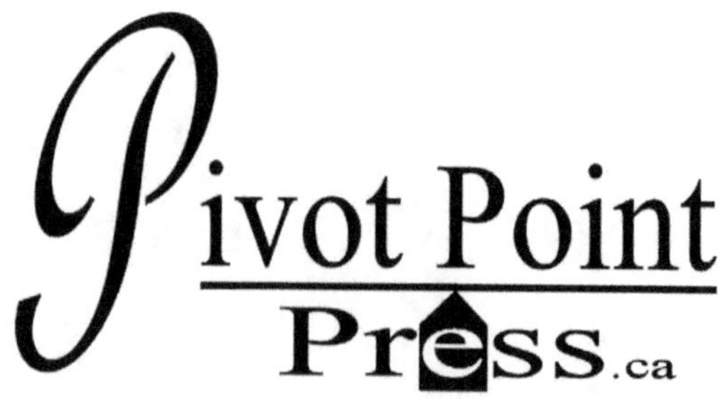

Publisher's Cataloging-in-Publication Data

Names: Godlewski, Paul, 1961- .

Title: Concussion. Brain on pause. How to hit play : a practical and illustrated guide to overcoming concussion, post concussion syndrome (PCS), and mild traumatic brain injury (mTBI) / Paul Godlewski, PT.

Description: Toronto, Canada : Pivot Point Press.ca, 2024. | Includes index and bibliographic references. | 55 b&w illustrations, including line drawings, pictures, tables, and graph. | Summary: Provides treatment information for those 13-65 (and their caregivers), in layman's language, for concussion issues: headaches, fatigue, vision problems, sleep disturbance, dizziness, balance problems, and sensitivities. Also provides age-appropriate resources on returning to study, play, and work; advice when it's best "not to go it alone;" and whom to consult.

Identifiers: ISBN 9781738327843 (hardcover) | ISBN 9781738327836 (pbk.) | ISBN 9781738327850 (ebook)

Subjects: LCSH: Brain – Concussion. | Brain – Concussion – Treatment. | MeSH: Brain Concussion – therapy. | Post-Concussion Syndrome – therapy. | BISAC: MEDICAL / Neurology. | MEDICAL / Evidence-Based Medicine. | MEDICAL / Sports Medicine.

Classification: LCC RC394.C7 G63 2024 | DDC 617.481 G--dc23

For Karol & Marie Christine Godlewski
&
For My Patients

Testimonials

Advance Praise for:
Concussion. Brain on Pause. How to Hit Play.

"The section on post-concussion dizziness is a fantastic primer for vertigo and dizziness in general. Excellent explanations are found within that are appropriate for the average reader. The descriptions of the rehabilitation exercises, when and how to do them, and how to progress them provide an effective pathway for those suffering from concussion-related dizziness."

Alex Osborn, BSC, MD, PhD. Specialist in Otolaryngology.

"Paul Godlewski's book has many essential elements to help those with a concussion or Persistent Post-Concussive Symptoms. It covers the most common issues such as: headaches, dizziness, and vision problems. It provides detailed and practical management strategies. An important and useful addition to patient education and self-care."

Alice Kam, MSCCH, MT, MD. Specialist in Physical Medicine and Rehabilitation.

"Paul Godlewski has written an excellent, comprehensive, user-friendly practical manual for concussed patients, particularly those dealing with concussion-related headaches. An essential asset for them, as well as a useful addition to many a clinician's tool kit."

Deborah Fisher, BA(Hons), MD, CCFP. Headache management consultant.

"A great guide for any patient trying to navigate a return to learning, work and play. The book's approach to getting back to activity is comprehensive. It shows the concussed person: how to take control, manage their symptoms, and build confidence, all for a safe and successful return to a fuller life. The book's examples highlight common challenges faced by patients and practitioners alike. It is a patient-centred approach that draws from both real-life experience and the most up-to-date practice recommendations."

Nathaniel Ibey, BSED, BA, MD, CCFP (SEM). Dip. Sport Medicine.

"It is so refreshing to read a guidebook that not only outlines simple, logical, and effective procedures to manage concussion symptoms, but also gives those who suffer from concussion validation that their symptoms are real and hope that they can be helped. As a neuro-optometrist who specializes in the treatment and management of Post-Concussive vision deficits, I was pleased to read Paul Godlewski's book with its collaborative, holistic approach to care, rooted solidly in neurology and evidence-based procedures. I will definitely be recommending this book to my patients!"

Angela Peddle, BSCs, OD, FCOVD. Founder of Elite Vision Therapy Centre & Neuro-Visual Consultants.

"Having spent most of my 37-year career as a Physiotherapist working in the world of concussion rehabilitation, one of the most significant challenges that individuals with concussion face is a lack of accurate knowledge concerning their recovery. This important book by Paul Godlewski provides the individual with the knowledge and resources to assist in managing their symptoms and navigating the best possible recovery from their concussion. Knowledge is power and this book is powerful. It should be in every concussed person's library... I can't wait to pick up a copy - I'll be recommending copies for my patients for sure."

Bernard Tonks, BSC (PT), FCAMP, CVRT, PT Reg (B.C.). Dizziness and Balance Rehabilitation Clinic.

"In easy-to-understand everyday language, Paul Godlewski has created a comprehensive guidebook for how best to recover from a concussion or Post Concussion Syndrome. From my perspective as a psychotherapist, registered social worker, he deals well with the combined physical, psychological and social challenges that many concussed persons encounter on their road to recovery. His use of first-person narration draws you in and makes you feel like he is speaking directly to you. His extensive knowledge and experience shine through and provide hope for patients and their loved ones. The author references the latest research, uses practical cases and metaphors to justify the book's recommendations and to explain complex medical matters. These, married together with his wonderful sense of humour, make for an engaging read."

Patricia Bain, BSW, MSW, SW Reg (Ont.). Bain Counselling & Psychotherapy Services.

"*Concussion. Brain on Pause. How to Hit Play* offers a thorough guide through the labyrinth of life after Concussion and Post Concussion Syndrome. This empowering self-help resource combines the author's clinical experience with real-life stories and evidence-based science, providing a roadmap for recovery. The book presents exercises and practical strategies to combat daily challenges for all those rebuilding post-injury. A great read for anyone seeking strength, understanding, and a path forward."

Bonnie Cai-Duarte, BSC (PT), MSc, PT Reg (Ont.). UHN-TRI's L.E.A.P. Program for Brain & Spinal Cord Pain.

"With the help of Paul's book, you can learn to pace and plan like a pro, only needing to seek out a clinician if you are struggling. Following a concussion or Persistent Post-Concussive symptoms, this is an indispensable resource for anyone trying to get back to what they want to do, or have to do."

Elise Kopman, BHSC, MSC (OT), OT Reg (Ont.). Lifemark Health Group.

Google Reviews from Former Patients for: *Paul Godlewski, Concussion PT treatments*

"...I am a healthcare professional, and I work on a Neurological Rehab Inpatient Unit... Paul Godlewski is very, very well respected among the physiotherapy community for his work in concussion and vestibular rehab, and now I can attest to it as well. His assessment was thorough, he provided detailed education and handouts about different aspects of my recovery, and he made a customized treatment plan. Paul looks at patient's injuries holistically, and recommends other clinicians as appropriate (e.g., a sleep doctor, etc.). Also, he has a great rapport with his patients - he is funny, supportive and tough when he needs to be. Finally, he helped me to gradually return to work full-time and the activities I enjoy, and set me up for success. If I could give him 10 stars, I would."

Alana P.

"Paul Godlewski is clearly an expert at what he does. I'm a semi-pro soccer player and Paul really made a big difference in my recovery and return to play. Paul was able to identify and provide the kind of care I needed for a complex set of circumstances, including long-term vestibular loss and concussion. He was able to build a program for me that was geared towards my needs as an athlete. Paul's help was pragmatic and thorough. I recommend him very highly."

Ben L.

"I was diagnosed with a concussion in November 2022 after my son jumped on me and we bumped heads. It was so bad that noises affected me, my balance was off and I constantly felt like I had the lightheaded effect you get after blowing up a balloon. I couldn't sleep in my own room because the rustling of sheets was too much for my brain to handle. I needed earplugs to go grocery shopping and had to take many breaks. I had a hard time having conversations or handling new information... It took time, but I would say I am 90% back to what I was before... I know every concussion is different, but I just want to say that for me, Paul Godlewski was an instrumental part of me getting back to my life again…"

Karen F.

"…I saw Paul Godlewski after my concussion - he is very knowledgeable and a true expert in his field! His approach and therapy have provided me with significant improvement with my Post Concussion Syndrome. He is also very well connected and helped me build a team of practitioners to further help with my care. I wouldn't think twice about seeing Paul if you've experienced a concussion."

Nadine S.

"Paul is very thorough, detailed and keeps up to date on the latest research and cares about outcomes for his patients. I had two concussions within a 4-year period and both times Paul was able to make me feel comfortable, stabilize my concussion symptoms and return me to a functional state for work and living…"

Steve P.

Contents

Part 1: Only Your Brain Is Smart Enough to Heal Your Brain

Appendices

Test and exercise videos, etc.
featured in this book

Introduction

Fortunately for most, this injury results in symptoms a little more severe than a bump on the head. Such symptoms vanish almost as quickly as they came, leaving no trace. For others, it will result in functional limitations that can last for months. For a few less fortunate, it indelibly marks them, changing the course of their lives. Regardless, they all receive the same initial diagnosis. *Concussion*.

This is a self-help book about concussion, but with a difference. It's not just for those seeking relief from their concussions, but as well for those wishing to help those dealing with the affects of a concussion. A man involved in a motor vehicle collision looks for what he can do himself to alleviate his constant headaches. A mother looks for answers to how she can get her sports-injured son finally back to school. An adult child wants to know which clinician can best help her with her elderly mother's dizziness from a recent fall.

My book is written in simple, but not simplistic, language, with a bit of humour to help the medicine go down. It is structured to allow anything from a quick read, all the way to a deeper exploration of a specific issue. Step-by-step, I will show you how to resolve a concussion's most common symptoms: fatigue, sleep disturbance, light/sound sensitivity, headaches, vision issues, dizziness, and balance problems. Just as important, you will learn when "not to go it alone," and whom to consult. All this so that you can get back to what you need, or want, to do.

Okay, Let's Get Real. The Brain Is Extremely Complicated!

A while ago, I listened to a neurologist on the radio discussing the enormous amount of gobbledygook about the brain as represented in the media. To put neurologists' current understanding of the brain into stark relief, he said something like: *Look, we are getting pretty good at understanding how a single neuron works. Our knowledge of networks of up to ten neurons is coming along quite nicely, thank you. As for understanding how the 100 billion neurons in your brain work, well, let's just say that's a bit far off.*

That's it then, isn't it? Brains are far too difficult to understand. Close the book. We can't really do anything to help with brain injuries. Right? *Wrong!* In fact, we rely on the brain's amazing complexity and inborn capacities to heal itself. Nevertheless, the neurologist's point is a very good one. We are only just starting to understand the brain, and there is indeed a lot of poorly founded hype. In part, this book sets out to make you a more informed consumer of the various evidence-based treatment options out there.

Given our somewhat limited understanding of the brain, all who work in this field have to adopt a very humble, pragmatic approach. If you're depending on one or more clinicians (including the one writing this book) to "heal" your brain, you are going to be very disappointed. That's because the key player in your healing is *your brain*, and what you do with it. Your brain is really the team member that is doing the heavy lifting in your recovery. Clinicians act mainly as knowledgeable assistants to your brain, optimizing the environment to help the brain do its thing.

Persistent Post-Concussive Symptoms (PPCS) is the medical term favoured by most clinicians for any concussion symptom that lasts longer than one month from the date of injury. Later in the book, I will discuss why Persistent Post-Concussive Symptoms (PPCS) has supplanted the older term Post Concussion Syndrome (PCS). I will also explain why this change in terminology is important to the enhancement of your recovery (see Chapter 1).

Even given the complexity of the brain, there is already quite a lot we can offer to someone with a concussion or Persistent Post-Concussive Symptoms (PPCS) to hasten their recovery and help them feel more comfortable. Of all the approaches, one of the most important is your activities and exercise. When it comes to rewiring your brain (aka neuroplastic recovery), both your activities and exercises are very important. The brain uses these to direct its healing (see Chapter 2).

The Epidemic Called Concussion

In Canada, there are about 150,000 - 200,000 concussions annually.[1,2] In the United States, figures from the Center for Disease Control (CDC) state that in 2014 there were about 2.87 million Traumatic Brain Injury (TBI)-related emergency department visits, hospitalizations, and deaths. This statistic has risen by more than 50 percent from the previous 2006 figures. Even if some of this is a result of more concussion awareness, this is a huge increase.

Rates of emergency department visits per 100,000 population were highest among older adults (seventy-five years of age or older), then young children (birth to four years of age), closely followed by youths aged fifteen to twenty-four years. Respectively, falls, being struck or striking an object, and motor vehicle crashes were the most frequent causes of TBI-related emergency visits.[3] In an earlier document, the CDC calculated that 87 percent were treated in and released from emergency (most likely as a result of mild TBIs/concussions), 11 percent were hospitalized and discharged (most likely as a result of moderate to severe TBIs), and 2 percent died (most likely severe TBIs).[4]

Finally, the CDC estimates that mild traumatic brain injury (mTBI, aka concussions) account for at least 75 percent of all traumatic brain injuries (TBIs) in the United States.[5] All of these CDC numbers likely underestimate the total occurrence of TBIs in the US, as they don't account for those who did not get any medical care, those who had just doctor's office-based visits, or those who received care at a federal source (e.g., US military). Looking globally, it has been estimated that there are 69 million TBIs annually! [6]

The estimate is that a minimum 15 percent of first-time concussions go on to develop Post Concussion Syndrome (i.e., concussion-like symptoms lasting for three months or more). To use a back-of-an-envelope calculation, this means that, yearly, there are 22,500 – 30,000 cases in Canada, 320,000 in the US, and approximately 7,750,000 worldwide which result in longer-term symptoms and disability. These figures are staggering. It fully justifies the use of the term epidemic and demonstrates the need for prevention, quality concussion information, and evidence-based treatments.

The Need for This Book, and Who It Is Meant For

Why this particular book? After all, there are many wonderful books already available about concussions, such as Dr. Elizabeth Sandel's *Shaken Brain: The Science, Care and Treatment of Concussion*.[7] In addition, there are quite few good books with moving personal stories of how concussion and PPCS have affected a person, and how they have overcome their condition. See Sarah Polley's *Run Towards the Danger*. [8]

What is missing in many of these books is what you can do for yourself or for a loved one with a concussion or PPCS. In my experience, what these concussion/PPCS patients and their caregivers need most is straightforward, evidence-based information. For many, this is very hard to come by due to their location, lack of medical coverage, and/or income. This book is written to bridge this information gap with a partially do-it-yourself (DIY) approach to concussion management, aimed at the average person (aged thirteen to sixty-five years of age) suffering from either a concussion or PPCS, along with their loved ones trying to find ways to help them. It's written as a practical how-to manual full of information, advice, and exercises. Though they are very useful, this work is not meant to be a medical book written by multiple experts in their fields. It's designed instead as a relatively easy read—hopefully amusing at times—that offers you practical information you can apply immediately.

Do-It-Yourself (DIY) Versus Professionals. Is It One or the Other?

Depending on your needs, the answer is quite often no— it's both. Taking ownership of your condition is empowering and will lead to a much better recovery. What you do matters enormously. In fact, your active involvement is *absolutely key* to your getting better!

A Roadmap for This Book

<u>Part 1</u> - Only Your Brain Is Smart Enough to Know How to Heal Itself (chapters 1-2)
These first two chapters provide you with the general principles on how the brain can heal itself and the things you can do to help it along. They give you important information you will use repeatedly to hasten your recovery.

<u>Part 2</u> - How to Help the Brain Help Itself (chapters 3-7)
This part of the book takes a symptom-by-symptom approach for the most common and troublesome concussion/PPCS symptoms. Bear in mind that a given symptom can come from multiple sources. For example, headaches can come from the trauma to the brain, from problems related to your vision, and/or from neck issues. Therefore, you may need to dip into a couple of different chapters in order to best overcome a particular symptom. Where necessary, I will direct you to other chapters in the book.

<u>Part 3</u> - How to Get Back to What You Want and Need to Do (chapters 8-9)
Once your symptoms are better controlled and reduced, this part of the book provides direction on how to safely get back to your regular activities.

The Time Phases of Recovery

Recovery can be broken down into two phases. As time and recovery advance, so too do the goals and activities that can be undertaken.[9,10] In general, earlier demands you impose on the brain need to be lighter. As recovery continues, *potential* inflammation (see chapter 1) is thought to lessen; activities can therefore become somewhat more aggressive. Some individuals with mild concussions will zoom through all the stages and get back to normal activities soon. Still, caution needs to be employed. A lack of symptoms does not necessarily mean the concussion is fully healed. The brain can still be irritable, prone to flare-ups.

Acute Phase (0-4 weeks) [10]
The goal: to help relieve your symptoms, settle *potential* inflammation, and restore the brain to a more balanced state (aka, restore homeostasis). In general, during the early days of a concussion, most of the information you will need can be found in chapters 1-4. It will make the most sense if you read this information in the order of these initial chapters. During this acute stage, the emphasis for treatment is on:
- Education about the condition, your own role in recovery, and how best to resume activity (see chapters 1 and 2).
- Concussion-tailored cardiovascular exercises to rebuild energy (see chapter 3).
- Methods for keeping symptoms below a certain threshold to hasten recovery and avoid chronicity (see chapters 3 and 4).
- Interventions to improve sleep and reduce fatigue (see chapter 4).
- Managing light and sound sensitivity (see chapter 4).

- For faster recovering concussions, a graduated return to activity (see chapters 8 and 9).

If your dizziness is lasting longer than ten days post-injury, it's recommended that you undergo formal cervicovestibular rehabilitation (e.g., see a physiotherapist/ chiropractor trained in both manual neck therapy and vestibular rehabilitation therapy).[10]

<u>Persistent Phase</u> (4-plus weeks) [10]
The goal: to assist your brain in healing via potential inflammation reduction and begin neuroplastic recovery. During this stage, the emphasis for treatment is on:
- Principles to hasten recovery (see the latter part of chapter 2).
- A symptom framework more appropriate for a persistent condition (see chapter 3).
- Interventions to reduce headaches, including neck therapies (see chapter 5).
- Managing dizziness, nausea, and balance problems (see chapter 6).
- Interventions to overcome visual dysfunction (see chapter 7).
- A gradual return to activity (see chapters 8 and 9).

If your symptoms are not improving or are worsening, it may be necessary to consult other professionals (see the individual chapters for examples of "when not to go it alone"). Thereafter, if your symptoms are not improving or are worsening, a multidisciplinary approach may be needed. This can be done in one integrated health facility, if available, or through multiple experienced community practitioners communicating with one another.

The Chapters' Common Components and How to Take Advantage of Them

While not all the chapters will include all these components, most will. Their order will vary depending on the needs of the given topic. However, most often, you'll find them organized in the following order:

Cheat Sheets

Individuals with concussions—especially those newly injured—will have a very limited endurance for reading and thinking. This section will help you to dip, skim, and skip as you need. In the very early days, it's recommended to have someone else read to you in small, bite-sized pieces. Don't feel you have to read this book cover to cover. Design your reading experience to suit your needs.

Concussion Stories

Each chapter starts with a story designed to help you and your loved ones understand how people experience and recover very differently from a concussion or PPCS. Recovery times vary greatly. They can be quite short, medium in duration, or quite long. These stories are an amalgamation of the many concussion patients I have seen over the years (i.e., they do not describe the experiences of any specific person).

The generally longer recovery periods quoted in many of my stories reflect the fact that most of the patients consulting me were having more persistent symptoms. However, many concussed individuals will recover far faster. This kind of patient rarely seeks out a clinician like me.

Deep Dive

Occasionally, I've selected topics for a closer examination. If you're curious, these boxed areas will give you greater insight into symptoms that may be giving you particular problems. They often give the foundational theory behind the treatments and exercises being recommended.

Tests to See if a DIY Approach Will Likely Help

Testing is the key is to doing the exercises that will really make a difference for you. Many chapters provide you with some tests you can carry out on yourself (sometimes with help from a family member/friend).

A Do-It-Yourself (DIY) Approach to Relieving Symptoms

Where appropriate, I provide practices and exercises that the person with a concussion or PPCS can do themselves. These are given both to help reduce your symptoms and restore your ability. You will find some of the tools you need to do these exercises in the Appendices.

When Not to Go It Alone

Sometimes it is better, even necessary, not to go it alone. To this end, in Parts 2 & 3 I have given you examples of when it is best for you to consult a professional(s) and whom. In all cases, you should consult your family doctor (GP) as well.

References

Endnote references are documented here. The references I provide are those that I found most helpful. In terms of material, they offer the deepest dive, justifying my recommendations, giving credit where credit is due, and informing readers who want to explore a given topic in more detail.

The Evidence, Safety, and Limitations of This Book's Recommendations

Evidence-based practice was the most important part in putting together this book. I have therefore footnoted the sources from which I have drawn. The reality is that these are still very early days in our understanding of the brain and, therefore, its rehabilitation. As a result, a given therapy may have been only partially studied, or not studied at all. In the absence of clear research guidelines, this means that clinicians need to use other supplementary sources of information.

The reasons for treatments and my recommendations come from a ranking of four sources. Beginning with the most important, these are:
1. Scientific studies investigating concussion (mTBI): If footnotes are not provided, assume I am using one of the other approaches.
2. Our current, unfortunately still limited, understanding of neuroplastic recovery and how to promote it (see chapter 2).
3. Anatomical and/or physiological reasons.
4. My experience in clinical rehabilitation, along with the clinical experiences of those who initiated my learning about this fascinating topic (see acknowledgments). I have endeavoured to state when the recommendations are predominantly coming from me.

The field of physiotherapy varies by country. In Canada, physiotherapists are independent practitioners who assess and diagnose issues in the physical domains. For example, in the vision sphere (see chapter 7), oculomotor dysfunction can be assessed by a physiotherapist like myself. Retinal dysfunction, as an example, is beyond the scope of a physiotherapist's practice. As such, where I have reviewed areas that are outside my profession's domain, I use references to justify my statements.

Moreover, I have had the manuscript reviewed for accuracy by multiple clinicians from many different professions (see acknowledgements). If the reader needs more, I refer them to the appropriate profession(s) for a more in-depth examination of a certain issue. For example, I provide only general information on sound desensitization. If the reader would like more help, I direct them to an audiologist and/or psychologist for more detailed assessment and treatment.

When it comes to all medical interventions, a practitioner's primary concern must be: "First, do no harm" (Hippocrates). Fortunately, the vast majority of physically based rehabilitation treatments and recommendations, being conservative and non-invasive, are safe. However, with a few instances in this book (e.g., specialized cardiovascular treatment in chapter 3), I recommend you always *first* consult your family doctor, or an appropriate specialist, to get their approval before commencing a treatment.

Do not ignore these precautions!

No single book can hope to cover all aspects of concussions or PPCS and all the knowledge and experience of many different professions. I have limited myself to covering only the physically based treatments and strategies that you can use to help yourself. As a result, medication, diet and supplements, psychological counselling, and alternative therapies, though very useful and at times necessary, are beyond the scope of this book.

An Important Final Note

This book is not to be used to self-diagnose any kind of brain injury, including a concussion. If you think you may have sustained a concussion, go to your nearest emergency department (ER) as soon as possible, then consult your family doctor. In addition, the material covered should not be considered a replacement for proper medical assessment by certified medical clinicians.

Nevertheless, this book can act as a good supplement to their assessments and subsequent treatments. If there is a contradiction between the advice you are receiving from the on-the-ground qualified clinician and this book, opt for your clinician's advice, at least *initially*, as they are able to customize their treatments to your individual condition and circumstances.

References

1. Langer, L., Levy, C. and Bayley, M. 2020. "Increasing Incidence of Concussion: True Epidemic or Better Recognition?" *J. Head Trauma Rehabil*, 35 (1) E60-66.
2. Report of the Standing Committee on Health - Report 24. 2019. *Tackling the problem head-on: Sports-Related Concussions in Canada.* House of Commons, Canada 42nd Parliament, 1st Session.
3. Centers for Disease Control and Prevention. 2019. *Surveillance Report of Traumatic Brain Injury - Related Emergency Department Visits, Hospitalizations, and Deaths - United States 2014.* National Center for Injury Prevention and Control. U.S. Department of Health and Human Services.
4. Centers for Disease Control and Prevention. 2010. *Traumatic Brain Injury in the United States Emergency*

Department Visits, Hospitalizations, and Deaths 2002 - 2006. U.S. Department of Health and Human Services.

5. Centers for Disease Control and Prevention. 2003 *The Report to Congress on Mild Traumatic Brain Injury in the United States. Steps to Prevent a Serious Public Health Problem*. U.S. Department of Health and Human Services.

6. Dewan, M.C., et al. 2018. "Estimating the Global Incidence of Traumatic Brain Injury." *Journal of Neurosurgery*, 130, no. 4 (April), 1080 -1097. https://doi.org/10.3171/2017.10.JNS17352

7. Sandel, Elizabeth. 2020. *Shaken Brain: The Science, Care, and Treatment of Concussion*. Cambridge, USA: Harvard University Press.

8. Polley, Sarah. 2022. *Run Towards the Danger: Confrontations with a Body of Memory.* Toronto, Canada Hamish Hamilton a division of Penguin Random House.

9. Concussion Ontario. 2023. https://concussionsontario.org/. *Living Concussion Guidelines. Guideline for Concussion/Mild Traumatic Brain Injury and Prolonged Symptoms for Adults 18 years of age and older.* Ontario Ministry of Health. Ministry of Long-Term Care.

10. Patricios J.S., et al. 2023. "Consensus Statement on Concussion in Sport: The 6th International Conference on Concussion in Sport–Amsterdam. October 2022." *Br J Sports Med.* 57, no. 11 (June), 695–711. https://doi.org/10.1136/bjsports-2023-106898

Part 1

Only Your Brain Is Smart
Enough to Heal Your Brain

Chapter 1

Concussion and Persistent Post-Concussive Symptoms?

"What's in a name?" William Shakespeare

Cheat Sheet

1.1 What Is a Concussion?

I tease apart the latest definition of what a concussion is that emerged through consensus at the 2022 conference in Amsterdam.

1.2 How We used to Treat Concussions Versus How We Treat Them Now

Over the last few years, how we treat concussions has evolved greatly, and for the better. In this section, I explain what we currently think is the best way generally to deal with concussions.

1.3 Just How Long Is This #@^%^*! Concussion Going to Last?

Using my own experience as a clinician and some references, I provide answers for this tough question.

1.4 Persistent Post-Concussive Symptoms

For a long time, we have used the term Post- Concussion

Syndrome (PCS) for any issue lasting greater than three months following a concussion. However, many clinicians are now questioning if this is the correct term to use. Instead, they prefer to use a newer term, Persistent Post-Concussive Symptoms (PPCS). I explain what's in this new name PPSC and why it's important.

1.5 Is This a New Concussion or Just a Flare-Up?
Okay, something has happened, and there you are back with many strong symptoms. Based on my clinical experience, I give my take on these relatively frequent and frustrating relapses.

1.6 Brain Under Construction—Sorry for the Inconvenience
Other people's attitudes toward your concussion can make a difference to helping/hindering your recovery.

1.1 What Is a Concussion?

Here is the latest definition of concussion, which recently emerged through the consensus of a majority of clinicians (78.6 percent) at a 2022 conference in Amsterdam. Please note, this definition is for a sport-related concussion (SRC). However, most of this definition applies to concussions caused by other things.

Now, take a big breath. A sport-related concussion is:

"A traumatic brain injury caused by a direct blow to the head, neck, or body resulting in an impulsive force being transmitted to the brain that occurs in sports and exercise-related activities. This initiates a neurotransmitter and metabolic cascade, with possible axonal injury, blood flow change, and inflammation affecting the brain. Symptoms and signs may present immediately or evolve over minutes or hours, and commonly resolve within days, but may be prolonged.

No abnormality is seen on standard structural neuroimaging studies (computed tomography or magnetic resonance imaging T1- and T2-weighted images), but in the research setting, abnormalities may be present on functional, blood flow, or metabolic imaging studies. Sport-related concussion results in a range of clinical symptoms and signs that may or may not involve loss of consciousness. The clinical symptoms and signs of concussion cannot be explained solely by (but may occur concomitantly with) drug, alcohol, or medication use, other injuries (such as cervical injuries or peripheral vestibular dysfunction), or other comorbidities (such as psychological factors or coexisting medical conditions)." (Patricios, 2023, p. 697).[1]

The definition packs a great deal into just two paragraphs. Enlarging and explaining its key points is needed.

- According to the American Congress of Rehabilitation Medicine, the words "concussion" can be used interchangeably with the term "mild TBI," so long as brain imaging is found to be normal and there aren't good clinical reasons to use them differently.[2]

- By definition, all concussions are a form of a traumatic brain injury (aka, TBI). However, not all TBIs are concussions. There are five types of TBIs: (1) Concussion, (2) Extra-axial Hematoma, (3) Contusion, (4) Traumatic Subarachnoid Hemorrhage and (5) Diffuse Axonal Injury.[3]
- You do not need to be struck in the head or lose consciousness to get a concussion. Any force that is sufficiently strong and delivered in the right way to the body can cause a concussion. Also, concussions do not just happen during sports and exercising. Some other common sources of concussions are: falls, motor vehicle collisions, workplace injuries, domestic violence, and assaults.
- There can be various internal things going on inside a concussed brain, either individually or together. These may include damaged tissue in the brain, for example, axonal damage (damage to the brain's internal wiring system). However, such axonal damage may or may not be present. Other important processes are occurring as well (i.e., neurotransmitter and metabolic cascades, blood flow changes, and inflammation). These are too complex to go into in this kind of book.
- Symptoms can come on immediately or be delayed somewhat in their appearance.
- Fortunately, a large percentage of people experiencing a concussion for the first time will recover quickly and spontaneously (i.e., without the need for treatment). The picture is more complicated for those who have had multiple concussion diagnoses. Unfortunately, not all concussions go this way. For some, the symptoms can last for months. Finally, for a very small percentage of individuals, symptoms can be protracted, lasting for

years. Please note that I said the symptoms—*not* the concussion—can last for a varying amount of time. For more information on this important idea, see Section 1.4.

- Concussions are not visible on standard magnetic resonance imaging (MRI). Why is this? As noted above, not all concussions are thought to lead to axonal damage. With no structural damage, there is nothing to be seen on such standard imaging. That said, special imaging technology, mostly used for research (e.g., fMRI, tensor imaging, etc.) can sometimes "see" evidence of concussions.

If axonal damage has occurred, then why do standard MRIs still not see it? To answer this, you need to get a feeling for how very, very, very small your neurons (the brain's processing engines) and axons (the brain's wiring) are. Depending on the machine, the smallest thing a standard magnetic resonance imaging (MRI) machine can see is about 1 mm^3 (i.e., a cube measuring 1 mm x 1 mm x 1 mm).

Let's put that into perspective. A single drop of water has a volume of about 50 mm^3. So, 1 mm^3 is just 1/50 (0.02) of a drop of water. Even within this very small volume, there would be a minimum of 50,000 neurons. Via the axons, each such neuron connects, in turn, to around 6,000-10,000 other neurons—a minimum of 300 million connections! A concussion can therefore disrupt none, one, or multiple connections (i.e., axonal damage) in a given 1 mm^3 volume.

The neuroscientist David Eagleman put this more poetically by saying: "A typical neuron makes about ten thousand connections to neighboring neurons. Given the billions of neurons, this means there are as many connections in a single cubic centimeter of brain tissue as there are stars in the Milky Way galaxy" [4] (Eagleman 2011, p2). So, pat yourself on the back (not too hard!). To date, your brain is one of the most remarkable things we know of.

- There are twenty-three common symptoms with concussions.[5] These can be organized into:

<u>Physical Issues</u>
1. Headache
2. Head pressure
3. Neck pain
4. Nausea & vomiting
5. Dizziness
6. Blurred vision
7. Balance problems
8. Sensitivity to light
9. Sensitivity to noise
10. Feeling slowed down
11. "Feeling in a fog,"

<u>Cognitive / Metabolic Issues</u> (Some have both physical and mental contributions e.g., fatigue)
12. Difficulty concentrating
13. Difficulty remembering
14. Fatigue or low energy
15. Confusion
16. Drowsiness
17. Sleep disturbance

<u>Emotional Issues</u>
18. More emotional
19. Irritability
20. Sadness
21. Nervous or Anxious

<u>Autonomic Issues</u>
22. Abnormal heart rate
23. Excessive sweating

- There are other symptoms (e.g., tinnitus, vertigo, amnesia and apathy). However, some of these overlap with other descriptors, or are less common. Not all individuals with a concussion will have all these symptoms. The number of symptoms, their severity, and how long they last will vary greatly between one person and another, as well as between different concussion events for the same person.
- For a person to be diagnosed with a concussion, the individual does not have to have lost consciousness (or for that matter, sustained memory loss). That said, both of these things can happen as a result of a concussion.
- A concussion is a unique medical condition. Don't assume that associated symptoms, signs, and functional problems are coming only from other sources (e.g., drugs, alcohol, medication, cervical injuries, inner ear dysfunction, and psychological issues).

1.2 How We Used to Treat Concussions Versus How We Treat Them Now

Attitudes toward the management and treatment of concussion have undergone a number of shifts. Like a pendulum, the approach has swung from one extreme to another. The first approach was rather casual and brutal and was followed for years and years. Then everyone became very worried and swung hard and fast to the other extreme. So, the pendulum went from:

Oh, come on, you have just had your bell rung. Don't be such a wuss. Get back on the horse, to the game, to work! (i.e., DENIAL).

to

Oh my gosh, you've had a concussion! Go into a dark room and stay there until further notice! (i.e., CATASTROPHIZING).

Fortunately, most clinicians have moved to a third, more midway approach. A very brief period (24–48 hours) of physical and cognitive rest (including from screens) is valuable. Once newly concussed individuals are past this very early stage, they should try, *as tolerated*, to become gradually, increasingly more active.[1] These include activities of daily living, screen time, work, school, and leisure. For example: walking or using a stationary bike (see chapter 3).

Temporary increases in symptoms are very common, and expected. They do not mean that the activity is causing harm. However, while still concussed, it's best if you avoid activities, in degree or type, that give you more than a mild increase in your symptoms. In addition, that these symptoms only last for a relatively short period. Using a zero to ten-point symptoms scale (where zero is no symptoms and ten is the worst symptoms imaginable), "as tolerated" means an increase of no more than two out of ten points for less than an hour. If greater or longer, you should temporarily reduce your demands and, later, resume a slow, graduated return to activity.[6]

Finally, and importantly: while you are concussed, you need to avoid activities that have an increased risk of contact, collisions, or falls.[6]

1.3 Just How Long Is This #@^%^*! Concussion Going to Last?

Using some references [1, 7, 8] and my clinical experience, here are the answers that I share with my patients:

- Each concussion is unique. A subsequent concussion can be less or more severe than the previous one. In general, the more concussions you've had, and the longer it has taken for you to recover, the harder and longer a subsequent one may be to recover from.
- Because concussions are so variable, it is not really the best idea to compare yourself to anyone else with a concussion, or even a previous concussion event of your own.
- There are other factors known to increase the likelihood of more prolonged symptoms, such as: having a history of migraines, a learning disability, and a history of mental health issues or a family member having such a history. It is important to understand, though, that having these issues does not automatically lead to longer recovery times.
- The biggest predictor of longer recovery is the severity of a person's initial symptoms in the first few days after injury. This is particularly true if dizziness, visual problems, and/or mood issues are strongly present.
- Physical recovery most often outpaces both cognitive (i.e., thinking, reasoning, etc.) and emotional recovery.
- Females, particularly in their teens, seem to have a longer recovery period than males.
- The good news is that a very large majority of concussions will be over in ten to fourteen days with little or no aftereffect. About 80-90 percent of the general concussion population will be over their concussion within a three-month time frame.

Okay, here is some *possibly* not-so-great news:
- Full recovery is generally not achieved for individuals whose symptoms last beyond three years.

The problem with this latter statement is that it includes all those who have and haven't had adequate treatment, and those who have every kind of preexisting issue discussed. In my view, the only message you should take away is that more prolonged concussions need to be taken seriously. Acting early on is important. It matters what you do and the kind of help you receive.

1.4 Persistent Post-Concussive Symptoms

What's in a name? Well, in this case quite a lot. Medically, a "syndrome" is a particular type of condition that gives you similar symptoms, but which can come from many different things. This is the case with the use of the term Post Concussion Syndrome (PCS). There are nearly two dozen symptoms associated with both concussion and PCS. But the reason behind any one of these symptoms may be different for different people.

For a long time, we have used this term PCS for any issues associated with concussions lasting longer than three months. However, many clinicians are now questioning if this is the correct term to use. Instead, they prefer to use a newer term: Persistent Post-Concussive Symptoms (PPCS). There are four reasons for the use of PPCS over the old PCS:
- The name PCS implies that, three months on from the injury, a new condition called PCS suddenly emerges for some individuals. This has always seemed odd to most clinicians.

- If you accept that a new condition, PCS, emerges, there has been no clear, universally accepted diagnostic criteria for what PCS is and when it starts.
- While the symptoms undoubtedly came on with the original concussion, for any given individual, it is far less clear why these symptoms linger.
- Finally, the symptoms of concussion are very non-specific; those symptoms occurring well after your injury could be related to something other than the concussion now.

A classic example of this is headaches. It's already well-known that if an individual has a prior history of a headache condition (e.g., migraines), their headaches *may* worsen in severity and/or frequency following a concussion.[7] Also, an individual who almost never had headaches prior to the concussion can develop a headache condition after the concussion.[7]

Using the name PPCS rather than PCS, advocates say, leads to better treatment outcomes for individuals who have longstanding symptoms and functional problems. Looking at migraines as an example, they say just trying to generally treat this thing called PCS is not as useful as going to a professional who specializes in headaches and migraines.

Alternatively, or additionally, you may need to see a neuro-optometrist for functional eye issues (see chapter 7) or a physiotherapist or chiropractor for your neck (see chapter 5). This is the part of the puzzle a good concussion clinician will help you with, and why it is often best to combine any DIY approach with the counsel of an experienced clinician.

Any concussion-related symptom that lingers longer than a month is now considered persistent (i.e., greater than one month).[1] Studies report different results about how long symptoms can persist thereafter. One study noted that, a year on from the concussion, 50 percent of those surveyed reported they still had three or more symptoms, and 70 percent reported that one symptom was still significantly present.[9] An earlier study, which used the older term PCS (i.e., symptoms lasted more than three months), reported 11.4 percent to 38.7 percent of concussed individuals had persistent symptoms.[10]

Unfortunately, it's not easy to gauge if: (A) there is inflammation in the brain, (B) if there **is** inflammation, at what point does it usually resolve, and (C) if inflammation is present, is this a good and/or bad thing for the brain.[11] Until these factors are better understood, I believe it is best to be somewhat cautious.

Admittedly, while there are many things we don't understand about PPCS, clinicians are becoming better at treating it. The key is that PPCS treatments should not be just a continuation of concussion period treatments. The longer it is from the injury date, the more likely any *potential* tissue damage is healed and any *potential* inflammation, for good or bad, has resolved. The brain is therefore thought to be much less irritable as time goes on.

How do you put all this into practice? Using a combination of the older PCS and the newer PPCS approach, here is how I deal with symptom flare-ups and a return to activity:

- From the date of injury up to one month post injury, I am cautious in the degree to which my therapies and the patient's own return to activity are allowed to provoke higher and/or longer duration symptom flare-ups.

- After the one-month mark, many clinicians (including this one) believe the concussion period is officially over, and the individual is entering the PPCS period. During this period, the return to activity can be ramped up, *to a degree*, and we can become, up to a point (see chapter 3), less mindful of symptoms that are provoked.
- By the three-month mark, using the older PCS model, all clinicians believe it's safe to be more aggressive with a return to full activity.

The above are just general rules of thumb and need to be modified to the unique circumstances of each person. One size *does not* fit all. To aid you in customizing these rules to your particular situation, later on I will give you two different symptom-action frameworks, one for the concussion period and the other that is more appropriate for the PPCS period. Along with some other tools, these will help you to know how much to push yourself and when (see chapter 3).

If you continue to have problems beyond three months, we need to try to find out why. If you are struggling, the advice of a clinician(s) experienced in concussion management is especially useful. In some cases, what might be getting in the way of returning to normal function is an overly vigilant and protective nervous system. In addition, there may still be deficits (structural and otherwise) that cannot be overcome through the regular healing process. Instead, these need to be compensated for through the neuroplastic processes (see chapter 2).

1.5 Is This a New Concussion or Just a Flare-Up?

Let's say an incident has occurred that has significantly worsened your symptoms. Quite often, the incident is minor—your head is tapped by a child, say, or a pet. Prior to a concussion, such an incident would have hardly been noticed, or, if noticed, shrugged off. At other times, an individual will have a more major incident, like a fall, in which they may strike their head and flare their symptoms.

The question then arises: Have I sustained another concussion? This is a very tricky question to answer. I've been unable to find any good research into it. Nor does there seem to be a good explanation out there for why this seems to happen with such regularity to concussed individuals. If any researchers are reading this, this is a much-needed area of research!

For better or worse, you are left with my take on these two related questions. One observation I have made over the years is that the strength of the incident does not seem to be a good predictor of the flare-up's severity or how long it will last. I've seen clients who have experienced a major nosedive in their condition from a seemingly very minor incident. Other individuals have recovered quickly from what I was afraid was a new concussion. Thus, it's not possible to make blanket statements about whether or not something is a new concussion merely by understanding what caused the flare-up.

The experience of seeing many concussed individuals deal with such incidents has led me to conclude that the vast majority of these incidents are flare-ups, rather than a new concussion, and will take between two to four weeks to resolve back to the pre-flare-up level of symptoms and function. Regardless, recovery is greatly enhanced and safety ensured by treating the individual as if they have been re-concussed. This means enhanced levels of rest, especially in the first twenty-four to forty-eight hours, and a graduated return to activities. If it turns out there was no new concussion, this merely delays the individual for a bit. It will also likely enhance their return to the pre-flare-up situation. If they have been re-concussed, well then, the right course of action was taken.

Why does this seem to happen so often? Again, without research to advise, you're left with my take on this. I think it's for a number of reasons, including:

- Concussions are known to lead to a group of problems including reduced reaction time, poor balance, decreased depth perception, changes in midline perception, and vision problems (see chapters 6 and 7). Any one of these would make it more likely for an individual to do something that flares them up.
- One of your brain's main "reasons for being" is to protect you. Once the brain becomes injured, it becomes quite watchful for an extended period for any kind of threat to it. If it becomes re-irritated, it seems to overreact. In anticipation of tissue damage, I believe it revs up its healing and defensive systems, bringing back many of the initial symptoms like fatigue, fogginess, and light and sound sensitivity. In time, it "discovers" there was no real tissue damage, and so, metaphorically, sends the troops back to the barracks.

1.6 Brain Under Reconstruction—Sorry for the Inconvenience

Other people's attitudes to *your* concussion can make a big difference to helping or hindering your recovery. By other people, I mean the people that you deal with most of the time: family, friends, employers, and employees. I have often thought that having this lapel pin I designed would be useful. Humour often works best to inform others.

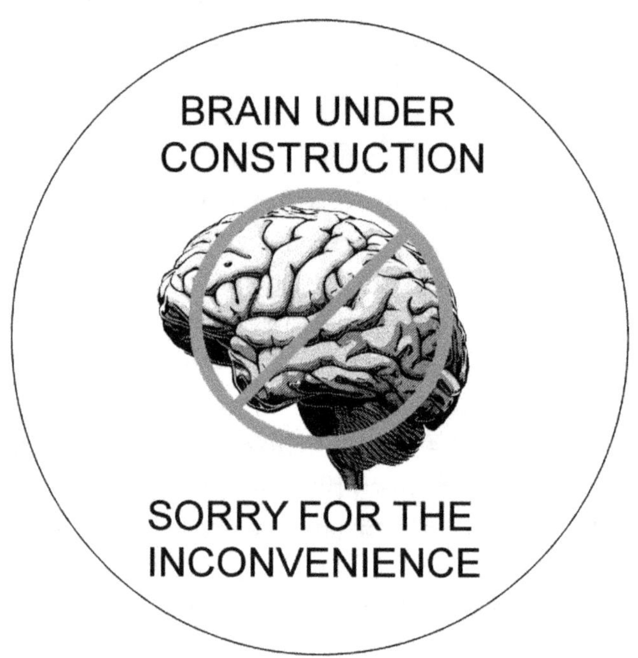

The following are education pieces designed to help the important people around you better understand. I am including both in the appendices for easier copying. First, not all that follows will apply equally to all individuals with this condition. It depends a great deal on what areas of the brain were affected, how long ago it happened, how severe the concussion/PPCS was, and how many concussions they have had.

I slightly modified the first education piece, "Nine Things to Consider," which is from the Amazing Brain Injury Survivor Support Group in Framingham, Massachusetts.[12] It is what I would call the "honey approach" to communication. If you need to hand out any of these information pieces, I suggest you try this approach first. It will also support your own experience that, no, this is not all in your head (well it is, technically, but…). It was written by individuals who have had concussion/PPCS.

I slightly modified the second education piece, "Nine Things NOT to Say," from St Joseph's Hospital Acquired Brain Injury Program, London, Ontario,[13] It is what I would call the "vinegar approach" to the education issue, when something a bit stronger is needed to get the message across.

Nine Things to Consider [12]
For a version you can copy, see Appendix A or
https://www.paulgodlewski.com/concussion-exercise-
tools-and-appendices/

- People with concussion/PPCS will often look better on the outside long before they have fully recovered. How they feel also changes greatly. They will have their good days and their bad days, their good moments and not so good ones.
- Individuals with concussion/PPCS can easily get physically and /or mentally fatigued. They will need much more rest than they are used to. Fatigue will make it hard for them to think and organize. Pushing too hard may lead to flare-ups and setbacks.
- The time to recover will vary greatly. Sometimes it will be mere days or weeks. Other times it may be much longer. Try not to compare one person with concussion/

PPCS with another. Recovery may also continue long after formal treatments have finished. They may or may not return to being exactly as they were. Expecting them to do so does not make it happen and puts a lot of stress on them for something generally not in their control.

- Allow people with concussion/PPCS to find their own words and follow their own thoughts. Doing this will help them rebuild their memory and language skills. Not remembering something does not mean that they don't care about it.

- Situations involving a lot of people in one place such as meetings, parties, religious services, and conferences can be very challenging for individuals with concussion/PPCS. They may resist going. This is because such individuals are often unable to filter and sort sounds and moving objects as well as before. If there is more than one person talking, they may not be able to follow the conversation. To have more time to understand what has been said, they may request you give them a pause or break.

- Individuals with concussion/PPCS may sometimes appear rigid in the way they do things, but repetition is a way for them to improve and will lead to better ways of doing things later.

- Acting out can be a sign of their inability to deal with a specific situation or built-up frustration from a number of things. They may be experiencing a lot of symptoms at the time, be overloaded by stimuli, tired, confused, and/or frustrated. Multitasking is challenging for all of us, but particularly for the brain-injured. Patience is the best thing you can give them.

- Tasks that are normally automatic or of little effort will take them much, much more effort and time. If they seem sensitive or emotional, it may be a reflection of the much greater effort it takes to do things. Help them by encouraging them. Try not to be too negative or critical. At that moment, they are likely doing the best they can.

- If a person with concussion/PPCS is having difficulty doing a task, doing it for them will not be constructive and will make them feel inadequate. If they appear stuck, asking what you can do to help may assist them to figure it out. Sometimes it may work best if you leave them to work things out on their own, at their own pace.

Nine Things NOT to Say [13]
For a version you can copy, see Appendix B or
https://www.paulgodlewski.com/concussion-exercise-tools-and-appendices/

Concussion is best thought of as a mild traumatic brain injury, not just a bump on the head. Brain injuries are confusing to people who don't have one. It's natural to want to say something, to voice an opinion, or offer advice, even when we don't understand. And when you care for a loved one with a brain injury, it's easy to get burnt out and say things in frustration.

Here are nine things you should avoid saying to someone recovering from a concussion/Persistent Post-Concussive Symptoms.

- *You seem fine to me.* The invisible signs of a brain injury—memory and concentration problems, fatigue, insomnia, chronic pain, depression, or anxiety—are sometimes more difficult to live with than visible disabilities. Research shows that just having a scar on the head can help a person with a brain injury feel validated and better understood. Your loved one may look normal, but shrugging off the invisible signs of brain injury belittles their struggles.

- *Maybe you're just not trying hard enough (i.e., you're lazy).* Laziness is not the same as apathy (lack of interest, motivation, or emotion). Apathy is common after a brain injury. Apathy can often get in the way of rehabilitation and recovery, so it's important to recognize and treat it. Certain prescription drugs have been shown to reduce apathy. Setting very specific goals might also help. Beware of problems that mimic apathy. Depression, fatigue, and chronic pain are common after a brain injury and can look like (or be combined with) apathy. Side effects of some prescription drugs can also look like apathy. Try to discover the root of the problem, so you can help advocate for proper treatment.

- *You're such a grump!* Irritability is one of the most common signs of a brain injury. Irritability could be the direct result of the brain injury, or a side effect of depression, anxiety, chronic pain, sleep disorders, or fatigue. Think of it as a biological grumpiness. It's hard to live with someone who is grumpy, moody, or angry all the time. Certain prescription drugs, supplements, changes in diet, or therapy that focuses on adjustment and coping skills can all help to reduce irritability.

- *How many times do I have to tell you?* It's frustrating to repeat yourself over and over, but almost everyone who has a brain injury will experience some memory problems. Instead of pointing out a deficit, try finding a solution. Make the task easier. Create a routine. Install a memo board in the kitchen. Also, remember that language isn't always verbal. "I've already told you this" comes through loud and clear just by facial expression.

- *Do you have any idea how much I do for you?* Your loved one probably knows how much you do and feels incredibly guilty about it. It's also possible that your loved one has no clue and may never understand. This can be due to problems with awareness, memory, or apathy—all of which can be a direct result of a brain injury. You do need to unload your burden on someone. Just let that someone be a good friend or counsellor.
- *Your problem is all the medications you take.* Prescription drugs can cause all kinds of side effects such as sluggishness, insomnia, memory problems, mania, sexual dysfunction, or weight gain—just to name a few. Someone with a brain injury is especially sensitive to these effects. But, if you blame everything on the effects of drugs, two things could happen. One, you might be encouraging your loved one to stop taking an important drug too early. Two, you might be overlooking a genuine sign of brain injury. It's a good idea to regularly review prescription drugs with a doctor. Don't be afraid to ask about alternatives that might reduce side effects. At some point in recovery, it might very well be the right time to taper off a drug. But you won't know this without regular follow-ups.
- *Let me do that for you.* Independence and control are two of the most important things lost after a brain injury. Yes, it may be easier to do things for your loved one. Yes, it may be less frustrating. But encouraging your loved one to do things on their own will help promote self-esteem, confidence, and quality of life. It can also help the brain recover faster. Do make sure that the task isn't one that might put your loved one at genuine risk—such as driving too soon or managing medication when there are significant memory problems.

- *Try to think positively.* That's easier said than done for many people, and even harder for someone with a brain injury. Repetitive negative thinking is called rumination, and it can be common after a brain injury. Rumination is usually related to depression or anxiety, so treating those problems may help break the negative thinking cycle. Furthermore, if you tell someone to stop thinking a certain negative thought, that thought will just be pushed further toward the front of the mind (literally, to the prefrontal cortex). Instead, find a task that is especially enjoyable for your loved one. It will help to distract from negative thinking and release chemicals that promote more positive thoughts.

- *You're lucky to be alive.* This sounds like positive thinking, looking on the bright side of things. But be careful. A person with a brain injury is six times more likely to have suicidal thoughts than someone without a brain injury. Some may not feel very lucky to be alive. Instead of calling it *luck,* talk about how strong, persistent, or heroic the person is for getting through their ordeal.

References

1. Patricios J.S., et al. 2023. "Consensus Statement on Concussion in Sport: The 6th International Conference on Concussion in Sport–Amsterdam. October 2022." Br J Sports Med. 57, no. 11 (June), 695–711. https://doi.org/10.1136/bjsports-2023-106898
2. Silverberg, N.D., et al. 2023. "The American Congress of Rehabilitation Medicine Diagnostic Criteria for Mild Traumatic Brain Injury." *Arch Phys Med Rehabil.* 104, no. 8 (Aug), 1343-1355 https://pubmed.ncbi.nlm.nih.gov/37211140/

3. Galgano M., et al. 2017. "Traumatic Brain Injury: Current Treatment Strategies and Future Endeavors." *Cell Transplant.* 26, 7 (Jul), 1118-1130. https://doi.org/10.1177/0963689717714102

4. Eagleman, David. 2012. *Incognito.* Toronto, Canada: Penguin Canada.

5. Patricios J, et al. 2023. *Sport Concussion Office Assessment Tool 6- SCOAT 6. For Adults & Adolescents (13 years +).* Br J Sports Med 57, no. 11 (Jun)

6. Leddy J.J., et al. 2023. "Rest and Exercise Early After Sport-Related Concussion: A Systematic Review and Meta-Analysis." *Br J Sports Med* 57, no. 12 (Jun): 762-770. https://doi.org/10.1136/bjsports-2022-106676

7. Concussion Ontario. 2023. https://concussionsontario.org/. *Living Concussion Guidelines. Guideline for Concussion/Mild Traumatic Brain Injury and Prolonged Symptoms for Adults 18 years of age and older.* Ontario Ministry of Health. Ministry of Long-Term Care.

8. Langer L.K., et al. 2021. Prediction of Risk of Prolonged Post-Concussion Symptoms: Derivation and Validation of the TRICORDRR (Toronto Rehabilitation Institute Concussion Outcome Determination and Rehab Recommendations) Score." *PLoS Med* 18, no. 7 (Jul), e1003652. https://www.doi.org/10.1371/journal.pmed.1003652

9. Machamer, J., et al. 2022. "Symptom Frequency and Persistence in the First Year after Traumatic Brain Injury: A TRACK-TBI Study." *J. Neurotrauma.* 39, no. 5 (Mar), 358-370. https://www.doi.org/10.1089/neu.2021.0348

10. Voormolen, D.C., et al. 2018. "Divergent Classification Methods of Post-Concussion Syndrome after Mild Traumatic Brain Injury: Prevalence Rates, Risk Factors, and Functional Outcome." *J. Neurotrauma* 35(11):1233-1241. https://www.doi.org/10.1089/neu.2017.5257

11. Patterson, Z.R. and Holahan, M.R. 2012. "Understanding the neuroinflammatory response following concussion to develop treatment strategies." *Front. Cell. Neurosci.* 6, no. 58 (Dec), 1-10.

https://www.frontiersin.org/articles/10.3389/fncel.2012.0
0058/full
12. Modified from the "Amazing Brain Injury Survivor Support
    Group, Framingham, MA." Cited in McGuire, S. 2014 PT
    Postgraduate course: "Concussion Management
    Workshop." Bridgepoint Heath, Toronto, Ontario.
13. Modified from one used St Joseph's Hospital Acquired
    Brain Injury Program. Cited in McGuire, S. 2014. PT
    Postgraduate course: "Concussion Management
    Workshop." Bridgepoint Heath, Toronto, Ontario.

Chapter 2

Guiding Principles for Treatments

"Any man could, if he were so inclined, be the sculptor of his own brain." 1904

"In adult centres the nerve paths are something fixed, ended, immutable. Everything may die, nothing may be regenerated." 1913
Santiago Ramón y Cajal

Cheat Sheet

2.1 A *Very Brief* History of Neuroplasticity

The concept of neuroplasticity has been around for a lot longer than most know. But it was only in the 1990s that the tide turned, and it became more universally accepted.

2.2 What Is Neuroplasticity?

Though neuroplasticity is a good thing, for the most part, it has its limits. Understanding this concept better may help you be realistic about how and when it can help you.

2.3 The Dark Side of Neuroplasticity

Examples of where neuroplasticity "breaks bad"

include: nerve injury in the body, amputations and phantom limb pain, chronic pain conditions, and addictions.

2.4 The Grey Side of Neuroplasticity
The neutral or grey side of neuroplasticity informs us the most about the reasonable limits of what neuroplasticity can do, and when.

2.5 The Light Side of Neuroplasticity
Neuroplastic changes in the brain are happening constantly, from blink-of-an-eye events to those that take decades. Fortunately, most of these changes are of huge benefit.

2.6 Treatment Guides to Promote Better, Faster Healing
In this final section, I outline principles found in scientific literature, along with my own experience to encouraging healing.

2.1 A *Very Brief* History of Neuroplasticity [1]

The two quotes at the start of this chapter show how long the idea of neuroplasticity has been around, and how two distinctly different ways of thinking about the nervous system have fought for dominance. Strangely, these two contradictory statements came from the same man, Santiago Ramón y Cajal. He is considered the grandfather of modern neurology.

In the first quote, he seems very optimistic about the capacity of the brain to change and our ability to influence it in any way we like. It is obvious from the second quote that Ramón y Cajal did a complete about-face in his thinking. He became convinced that, once infancy and early childhood are over, our brain's capacity is completely set and rigid, like dried concrete. For a very long time, this way of thinking dominated neuroscience and neurology. Everyone seemed to accept that the brain was not able to physically adapt or change past the early stages of our lives. Sort of a what-you-see-is-what-you-get kind of thinking.

In 1949, things began to change. Psychologist Donald Hebb hypothesized that memories in brains are formed by strengthening connections between neurons. He coined a now famous phrase: *What fires together, wires together.* In other words, the more often two neurons stimulate each other electrically, the stronger the physical connection between them will become.

But it was not until 1998 that the final nail was driven into the coffin of the long-held Ramón y Cajal dogma that the brain is fixed. Peter Eriksson and colleagues found that new cells are generated in relatively small quantities in an adult human's hippocampus. The hippocampus is known to be a very important component in the brain's ability to learn and form memories.

2.2 What Is Neuroplasticity?

In scientific literature, there are complex definitions of neuroplasticity.[2] But for our purposes, we can keep this explanation fairly simple and straightforward. "Neuro" is used for anything to do with the nervous system. *"Plasticity"* refers to something being flexible/malleable.

Putting these two parts together, all neuroplasticity really means is that the nervous system is not fixed but has the capacity to change. Neuroplasticity is a capacity that the entire nervous system possesses. Unfortunately, neuro-plasticity is often portrayed now as having some kind of mystical property. While neuroplasticity does have the capacity to change the whole nervous system, it is not magic! It has its limits; some we know, and likely many more waiting to be discovered.

Like many other readers, I was very much taken by books [3,4] by the psychiatrist Dr. Norman Doidge, particularly his 2015 book, *The Brain's Way of Healing: Remarkable Discoveries and Recoveries from the Frontiers of Neuroplasticity*.[4] Dr. Doidge's books made me further appreciate neuroplasticity's huge potential for all forms of neurological healing. I am even more indebted to the 2016 book *Neuroplasticity*,[1] by neuroscientist Dr. Moheb Costandi, for expanding my clinical understanding of neuroplasticity's long history (see above), and both its good and not-so-good sides.

Understanding neuroplasticity helps us form a better, more realistic picture of its true potential. Revelations from Dr. Costandi's book, combined with working for many years with concussed and vestibular patients, have revealed to me that neuroplasticity is no less miraculous but far less simple than I once thought. Dr. Costandi's book made me realize that neuroplasticity has three personas. Taking inspiration from George Lucas's idea of the "Force," I like to think of them as the dark, grey, and light sides.

2.3 The Dark Side of Neuroplasticity

I will very briefly review some examples of its dark side.[1]

<u>Peripheral Nerve Injury</u> (i.e., the nerves of the body, not the brain or spinal cord)
When a nerve in the body is seriously damaged or cut, it has to rebuild itself, finding its way via neuroplasticity from the spinal cord all the way back to its target (e.g., your muscles). Unfortunately, sometimes these new nerves "get lost" in the maze of tunnels along the way.

<u>Phantom Limb Syndrome</u>
When someone has had a limb amputated, they can at times continue feeling sensation from the absent limb. Sensations range from the mild, such as a feeling of pressure, through the odd, where they feel their limb is still moving, to the severe, such as burning or stabbing pains. Neuroplasticity is thought to play an important role in phantom limb pain.

<u>Chronic Pain</u>
In chronic pain, the pain continues for months, years, or, unfortunately, sometimes indefinitely after the injury has healed. Neuroplasticity is thought to maintain the persistence of this pain.

<u>Addictions</u>
The reward systems of our brain are an important part of what motivates us to do what we need to survive and prosper. Addictive drugs *"neuroplastically"* take over the brain's beneficial teaching system. An addict "learns" in error that the consumption of the drug substances is a good thing, when it is anything but good for them.

2.4 The Grey Side of Neuroplasticity [1]

In some ways, the grey side gives us more clues about the reasonable limits of neuroplasticity than either the light or dark side. Four examples of the grey side of neuroplasticity are: [1]

Critical Time Periods

From observation and experiments, we know there is a critical early period in the lives of mammals (including us) for the development of certain capabilities, like proper vision. Miss this window, or receive inadequate stimulation, and it will be much harder, if not impossible, for the individual to gain this sense capacity. That is why you can't just give new eyes to a blind person and expect them to see. In concussions to a degree, and particularly for PPCS, as more time passes, the going gets tougher and the gains that can be made are less significant.

Recovered Capacity Can Sometimes Be Less

Neuro-physiotherapists routinely work with patients who have sustained strokes. What individuals are able to regain through this rehab can be truly awe-inspiring. Still, once recovered, these individuals will often suffer long-term reductions in the quality of their movements and endurance. For example, their final ability to walk may be less smooth than before the stroke, and they may not be able to walk for as long.

The message here is that neuroplastic recovery sometimes restores the patient completely to the level of function prior to the injury, but can also, at times, only restore them in some areas to a partial level of their former capacity. The very good news is that the vast majority of concussion patients will recover fully. Sometimes this will take a shorter amount of time, sometimes longer, but in the end, most recover. Nevertheless, some patients can experience lingering symptoms, sometimes significantly so, that last longer than a year.

Individual Neuroplastic Capacity

Both your individual genetic profile and your environment will have profound effects on how much neuroplastic recovery you can get from a given injury. How well you do, therefore, cannot be compared to anyone else's speed and degree of recovery. Brain injury and its recovery are unique to the individual.

Neuroplasticity and Aging

There is somewhat contradictory evidence about the effects of age (i.e., children versus teens versus middle age versus older individuals) on neuroplasticity. Typically though, age brings cognitive losses and a noticeable shrinkage in the volume of our brains over the years. This happens gradually, not all at once. While we decline, it is very important to realize people don't have an expiry date: there is no "I am so sorry, your brain is just too old to recover." Barring certain illnesses, the brain continues to learn and adapt throughout a person's life. Nevertheless, aging does slow this recovery and, depending on the individual and the injury, may reduce the final degree of recovery.

2.5 The Light Side of Neuroplasticity

As part of constantly learning and perceiving your environment and forming new memories, millions of connections (aka, synapses) in your brain are changed. Time frames for neuroplastic change span those taking less than a second all the way up to changes that take decades (e.g., for a brain to fully mature from an infant to an adult one). Here are some examples: [1]

Unfortunately, as the brain ages, it loses more and more cells. So much so that imaging later in life, as noted, often shows a shrinkage in the overall volume. However, older adults still manage to perform very well compared to younger individuals. How do they do this? Neuroplasticity to the rescue again. It is believed that the brain rewires gradually, bringing on more and more areas to do a given task. In addition, it is thought that there is an increasingly efficient use of what is left. All this to say that neuroplasticity is a normal and quite wonderful part of your brain's function. While it's a very important part of recovering from an injury (e.g., a concussion/PPCS), it doesn't just kick in when something goes wrong. Fortunately, it's happening all the time—mostly to your benefit.

2.6 Treatment Guides to Promote Better, Faster Healing

I will now discuss the guiding principles for the treatments I use in clinic and throughout this book. These principles come from two sources:

- Science's growing understanding of how neuroplasticity can be used to overcome many neurological conditions including concussion (mTBI)/PPCS. Unfortunately, it is still early days as to how we can use these properties for therapeutic ends.[1] That being said, there are some characteristics we already know about neuroplasticity that can be utilized to help patients. Only the principles coming from scientific studies are footnoted below.

- My own clinical physiotherapy practice includes rehabilitating four different types of patients. Each of these have unique aspects to their treatments. At the same time, they share similarities from which we can draw lessons. The four different patient groups are: those with vestibular pathologies (i.e., those with inner ear dizziness conditions), those with neurological conditions (concussion, stroke, peripheral nerve issues, etc.), those with orthopaedic issues (i.e., injuries or illness related to the muscles, joints, tendons, ligaments, bones, and the nerves that supply them all), and those with chronic pain. Each of these patient types have unique, non-translatable features. At the same time, I believe there are lessons we can draw from all these patient types to aid the treatment of concussion and PPCS patients.

It's important to acknowledge that my experience is just that: my take on the effective treatment of concussion and PPCS. In other words, it is only level four of the evidence hierarchy discussed in the introduction.

Nevertheless, knowing all these principles I believe will help you to heal better and quicker. I hope it will also make you more willing to do the hard work and put up with the repetitive and, let's face it, sometimes boring exercises outlined in this book.

Principles for Both Concussions and Persistent Post-Concussive Symptoms

The more often things happen together, the more strongly they become associated in the brain.[1-5] This concept originates from the psychologist Donald Hebb in 1949 when he said: "What fires together, wires together." [1] Because the brain is such a complicated network of connections spanning across the whole brain, this principle happens not just at the neuron-to-neuron connection but throughout the brain.

When the brain is carrying out a behaviour, things that happen in the brain at nearly the same time tend to strengthen their link with each other. Often this can be a very good thing for us, as it allows for future beneficial cooperation within the brain. But, as with all things to do with neuroplasticity, it is not always so.

Let's take a negative example. If a certain movement like turning your head causes you to feel dizzy, and at the same time this provokes anxiety, they can start to become associated in the brain. If each subsequent time you get dizzy you also get anxious, this linkage becomes stronger—so much so that it can even start to work the opposite way. Each time you get anxious, you may also start to feel dizzy. If a strong enough linkage has been forged, you will likely need the help of vestibular and Cognitive Behavioural Therapists (CBT), plus or minus medication from an MD, to help break down this linkage.

Repeat, Repeat, and Repeat! [5]
When it comes to recovery, repetition is key. Your brain is a great pattern finder. The more data you give it, and the more consistent that data is, the more it has the capacity to learn and adapt its internal process. A good way to think about neuroplasticity is that you are rewiring your brain. This rewiring is no easy task. It is going to take a lot of persistent work and effort. That is because this is not really something the brain likes or wants to do. Quite frankly, if it can get away with not putting in the energy to do this, it will. By doing these exercises over and over again, you are, in no uncertain

terms, instructing your brain to get on with the work, and you don't mean perhaps!

For Any Given Day's Activity or Exercises, More Is *Not* Better

While frequent repetition is needed, it is repetition over the longer haul, rather than on a given day.

Like overcrowding a party boat, more and more exercises or activity is *not* the best approach. Instead, as will be outlined in greater detail in chapter 3, a Goldilocks approach is best, especially during the earlier stages of a concussion's recovery. Quick fatiguing is a very common characteristic of many neurological conditions, including strokes. This principle also seems to play out in recovery of concussions and Persistent Post-Concussive Symptoms. At all stages of recovery, you need to find the right balance between activity/exercises and rest. Your brain needs enough energy to enable it to learn to fix its problems. An exhausted or stressed-out brain is incapable of learning.

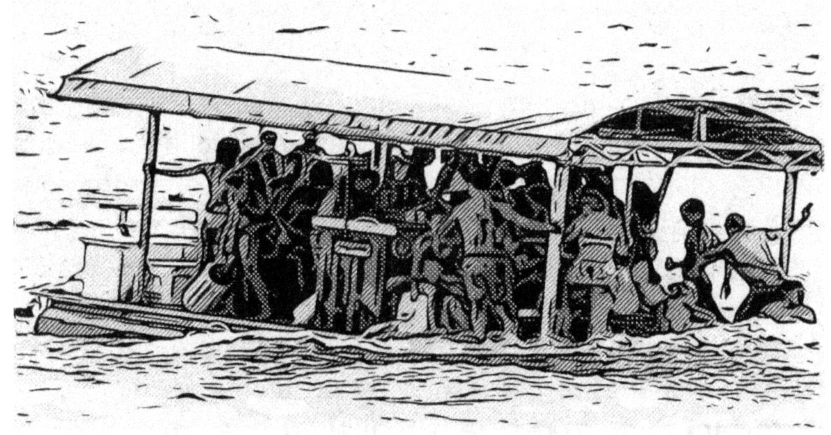

Adapted from a photograph taken July 4, 2014 by Lumina News. Permission for use given by Luma News: www.luminanews.com

In my exercises, I will ask you to do many repetitions of a given exercise, and I ask you to do them two to three different times a day. Doing more than I ask, however, will not give you a faster recovery. Please note, I am also not insisting on the third time, because concussion patients—and, to a lesser degree, PPCS patients—often struggle to do much of anything in the evenings (aka, the "sunset effect"). By that time, you have often run out of juice. It is therefore pointless to push doing more exercises. Far better to rest and pick up where you left off the next day.

<u>Start with Simple and Work Your Way Up</u> [5]
When you are trying to rehab the brain from an injury (e.g., a concussion), it's best to start by looking for problems at lower skill levels first and work up from these. Those with concussions and PPCS often struggle to carry out very basic vision and vestibular (i.e., inner ear) skills. They find they provoke symptoms and are generally harder and much more fatiguing to accomplish. However, without mastering these simpler skills, they will continue to have difficulty with high-order, integrated cognitive skills.

An example will help here. Visual skill steps can be arranged (starting with the lowest) as follows: visual acuity, visual field, fixating/unfixating, accommodation, global attention, versions, vergence, stereopsis, and visual perception. All these skills knit together to give you this amazing thing we simply call vision (see chapter 7). At this point, don't concern yourself with the details, as these skills may or may not be problems for you. The important thing to realize is that there are multiple skills underlying your vision.

Following a concussion, problems with any of these skills can act as a barrier to your recovery. That's because if any one of these lower skills is at fault, it will make the integrated upper-level skill called "visual perception" much more challenging for you. More challenging visual perception translates into greater difficulty learning or remembering and carrying out your activities of daily living (ADL), as well as increased fatigue.

To this end, most of the chapters in part 2 have simple tests for you to perform that will show you if you are or aren't struggling with one or another of these basic skills.

<u>The Early Fragility of Recovery</u>
One phenomenon I have noted is the fragility of early recovery. Patients have their good moments and bad ones, their good days and not so good ones. Rightly or wrongly, I think of this as a kind of battle for dominance between competing computer-like programs within the brain. Program A is how, up to the injury, they have always processed certain kinds of information. Program B is how the brain needs to process the information now that it has a concussion. The problem is that these programs seem to live together for a while after disease or injury. It's like they have to fight it out with one another to determine dominance. I find when concussed patients have had poor sleep or are ill, overtired from too much activity (see chapter 4), or stressed, they tend to have more bad moments or poor days.

<u>When Relearning a Skill, Initially Do So in a Less Distracting Environment</u> [1, 5]
You will learn quicker and make fewer errors if you work in a quieter environment that's not overly bright. In addition, try not to listen to music or engage in too much

multitasking. Later in the process, when you are more recovered, you will need to do the opposite—start bringing in more distractors and multitasking activities. This will better prepare you for resuming your normal activities in our busy, noisy, and chaotic world.

Don't Keep Doing the Same Old, Same Old [5]

Two neurotransmitters are released when you do something novel: acetylcholine and noradrenaline. Amongst other things, acetylcholine increases your attention to a task and your working memory. Noradrenaline also heightens your attention. Together they make it easier to pay attention to the given thing and to learn something new. The exercises in this book are arranged from easier to harder. It's important when you are ready to keep pushing forward, not just to keep doing the exercise level you have already mastered.

When You Succeed, Pat Yourself on the Back, and Don't Pay Undue Attention When You Don't [1, 5]

It turns out that the neurotransmitter dopamine is released when you succeed at some task or skill. Dopamine will induce in you a sense of pleasure. The pleasure, in turn, will make you want to succeed more (or fail less) in order to get more pleasure. The best way to reinforce this is to take note when you have accomplished something you couldn't do before, or could do but only at a lower skill level or quantity.

For example, when you started doing a balance exercise with your eyes closed, you could only manage to do so with your feet apart for ten seconds before you lost your balance. Now you can do it with your feet together for forty seconds. Good on you!

<u>However, You Need Both Success and Some Failure</u>[6]
Let's say you are trying to learn how to balance better on one foot (useful when dressing). If this task is so hard that you always end up quickly tipping over (potentially jarring yourself to boot), your system will learn little, and you may reinjure yourself. Likewise, if the task is a veritable breeze, your system will learn little. Therefore, I try to continually adjust my patients' exercises, either up or down, to target "medium hard" for them to do. I define "medium hard" as mostly success with some failure (but not to the point of falling, or jarring yourself!). You will also need to do this when exercising on your own.

<u>Learning the Same Message from Different Sensory Sources Works to Your Advantage</u> [7]
Researchers have found that learning is improved if people learn from multiple sensory sources. A vestibular (VRT) example from my own practice will help to illustrate this. Often, my patients experience dizziness because their left and right inner ears are not saying the same thing to their brain about where they are in space. Dizziness is the brain's symptom of confusion: *Gee, make up your mind, will ya? Am I here or am I **here**?!*

I will commonly give these patients a vision task called a gaze stability exercise, along with an eyes-closed balance exercise. Why is this? Because their brain is learning the same thing—in this case, that one inner ear is more reliable than the other, in two very different ways. One, through the gaze stability exercise (i.e., the vestibular and vision systems) and the other from the balance exercise (i.e., complex balance system). Each exercise reinforces the other and tells the brain that it has to change how it uses its inner ears.

<u>Physical Exercise Helps Cognitive Recovery</u>
(i.e., memory, thinking quality and speed, etc.) [1, 8, 9]
In both human and animal studies, it has been demonstrated that physical exercise, aerobic (for more info see chapter 3), and strength training improves cognition by the release of beneficial growth hormones called neurotrophins into the brain. These are thought to help your brain to heal and to improve memory.

<u>Brain Training, Like Physical Exercise, Also Enhances Cognitive Recovery</u> [1, 10]
There has been a lot of controversy surrounding cognitive exercise programs (e.g., Lumosity) which employ onscreen puzzles to improve cognitive capacities such as memory, multitasking, problem solving, etcetera. The promise was that somehow these programs would help the Boomers (like me) avoid or lessen the effects of an aging brain.

This didn't really happen, as the program's users improved their puzzle skills without necessarily retaining or increasing their capacity for real-life tasks. Unfortunately, this led many a clinician to throw the baby out with the bathwater and label all cognitive exercise as pointless. Research is now emerging that properly targeted training can be helpful in cognitive recovery.

<u>Reality Eventually Trumps Physio Exercises</u>
Performing real activities and tasks eventually becomes more important than all the exercises I might choose to give a patient. For example, take a concussion vision task called the "saccadic eye exercise." To be able to read this sentence, your eyes are moving accurately via a saccadic eye movement from one word to the next. To help concussion patients become better at this vision task, I

initially give them special saccadic eye exercises (e.g., Percon exercises, see chapter 7). Yet at the right time, it's important to get them to do real-life activities, such as light pleasure reading.

Why, you may ask, don't you go straight to doing the real-life tasks? The answer is that generally the injured individual needs to rebuild to a given capacity, first doing some simpler and easier exercise before they can tackle the real-life task (see above "Start with simple..."). Initially, reading is just too hard for some and brings on severe symptoms. Foundational exercises are therefore a very important run-up to the real-life applications. Nevertheless, these real-life tasks are more important. For this reason, when you feel up to it, most of my exercises in later chapters will give day-to-day activities you should start to do as well.

Principles for Persistent Post-Concussive Symptoms

I start using these principles about one-month post injury:

Avoid Too Much CAUTION Tape

Arguably, the most important purpose of your brain is to protect you from harm. The brain is always trying to draw lessons from what happens to you, particularly when it comes to things that threaten or injure you.

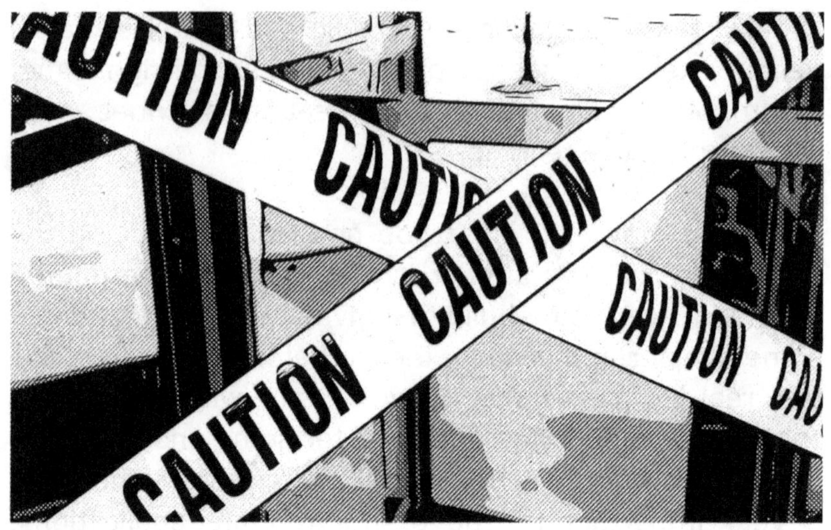

In this case, I think the brain sets up these caution tapes in the form of symptoms when you try to move past a given point. Unfortunately, sometimes the brain becomes overly cautious. It assesses the threat at a much higher level than the reality.

I find the brain is particularly inclined to do this overzealous caution-taping when the threat is to itself (go figure!)— like a concussion.

The solution to this is not to barge on regardless (tallyho, bungee jumping, here we come!). This approach just makes the brain very cranky and will get you a lot of strong, prolonged symptoms just to get the message across to you that "Really, I don't like that!" Instead, it's best to be persistent and to re-educate the brain about the reality of a given task, not to overly provoke its fears about the activity. Also, while it's likely that the brain is partially right in its assessment, it needs to bring its assessment into better alignment with the real world, and your need to work in that world. Again, I am not advocating engaging in risky behaviours where there is greater likelihood of you jarring or re-concussing yourself.

Don't Draw Conclusions from Too Little Evidence
When it comes to PPCS, I always instruct my patients not to draw too much from how they react to a new activity. For some reason, PPCS patients tend to respond badly to novelty, both new tasks and new environments. However, if they do the same thing again, they very often react less strongly. By the third time, sometimes they are not really reacting at all to the situation. I tell my PPCS patients that they need to be like scientists observing themselves. All things being equal, if, by the third time, their brain is still squawking at them about that task, it's time to respect its wisdom, leave off, and try it again later.

Consolidation Periods
During a slight upward or downward trend in the stock market, it's common for the financial market to go into a consolidation phase. That is, it simply persists in what it is doing, neither going dramatically up nor dramatically down. On occasion, I have noted the same in my PPCS patients. I don't really know what is going on during these periods, only that great patience is needed. I like to think that the brain is saying, "Look, I have a lot of rewiring to do here. Give me some space! When I am ready, I'll start improving again." These periods are frustrating to all, especially the patient, as they become fearful that this is as good as it's going to get. The answer to this is usually: "Stay calm, and carry on."

Gather Your Recovery While You May [1,2]
In concussions, to a degree, and particularly for PPCS, the going gets tougher as time passes, and the gains

made less significant (see above "critical time periods"). This is why I tell my patients not to procrastinate but to work as diligently as they can, as soon as they can. Although the window of recovery is open for quite a long time, it doesn't seem to remain so indefinitely.

<u>Different Strokes for Different Folks</u>
Neuroplastic capacity is very individual. The ability of your brain to rewire depends on so many factors. These include (in no particular order):
- your age;
- your gender;
- the severity of your injury;
- what areas of the brain are affected;
- how long ago the injury was;
- the number of concussions you have had;
- your underlying health status;
- your psychological coping capacity; and
- your genetic profile.

For this reason, you should not compare yourself with how other concussed people are doing, or what they have done, or even how you did the last time you had a concussion. Concussions and PPCS are like snowflakes; they are all different.

References

1. Costandi, Moheb. 2016. *Neuroplasticity.* Cambridge, USA. The MIT Press.
2. Cramer, S.C., et al. 2011. "Harnessing Neuroplasticity for Clinical Applications." *Brain* 134, pt. 6 (Jun), 1591–1609. https://doi.org/10.1093/brain/awr039

3. Doidge, Norman. 2007. *The Brain That Changes Itself: Stories of Personal Triumph from the Frontiers of Brain Science.* New York, USA. Penguin Books

4. Doidge, Norman 2015. *The Brain's Way of Healing: Remarkable Discoveries and Recoveries from the Frontiers of Neuroplasticity.* New York, USA. Penguin Books.

5. Nahum, M., Hyunkyu Lee, H., and Merzenich M.M. 2013. "Principles of Neuroplasticity-Based Rehabilitation." *Progress in Brain Research.* 207, 141-71. https://doi.org/10.1016/B978-0-444-63327-9.00009-6

6. Engineer, N.D., et al. 2012, as cited Nahum, M., Hyunkyu Lee, H., and Merzenich M. M. (2013) Principles of Neuroplasticity-Based Rehabilitation. *Progress in Brain Research.* 207, https://doi.org/10.1016/B978-0-444-63327-9.00009-6

7. Su, Y. S., Veeravagu, A., and Grant, G. 2016. "Neuroplasticity after Traumatic Brain Injury." in Laskowitz, D. and Grant, G. (Eds.) *Translational Research in Traumatic Brain Injury.* (Chapter 8 pp 1-12). Boca Raton, USA. CRC Press /Taylor and Francis Group.

8. de Sousa Fernandes, M.S., et al. 2020. "Effects of Physical Exercise on Neuroplasticity and Brain Function: A Systematic Review in Human and Animal Studies." *Neural Plasticity.* (Dec), 1-21. https://doi.org/10.1155/2020/8856621

9. Hötting K, and Röder B. 2013. "Beneficial effects of physical exercise on neuroplasticity and cognition." Neurosci Biobehav Rev. 37, no. 9 Pt. B (Nov), 2243-57. https://doi.org/10.1016/j.neubiorev.2013.04.005

10. Mahncke, H. W., et al. 2021. "A Randomized Clinical Trial of Plasticity Based Cognitive Training in Mild Traumatic Brain Injury." *Brain.* 144, no. 7 (Aug), 1994–2008. https://doi.org/10.1093/brain/awab202

Part 2

How to Help the Brain to Help Itself

Chapter 3

Concussion's Energy Crisis and Fatigue

"There is fatigue so great that the body cries, even in its sleep." Martha Graham

---

Cheat Sheet

3.1 How Zara Overcame Fatigue

Zara sustained a concussion from a fall from her bike. She initially struggled with headaches, neck pain, and fatigue. All were largely overcome by her own efforts, along with some key clinical sessions.

3.2 Energy, the Final Frontier

In large part, your energy level will determine the level and severity of your symptoms, and how fatigued you feel. Managing your energy level is also key to your healing.

3.3 Deep Dive: The Concussed Brain's Energy Crisis

This first deep dive provides a more detailed look at the underlying causes of low energy in the concussed and Persistent Post-Concussive Symptoms (PPCS).

3.4 To Rest or Not to Rest, That Is the Question

What is and isn't rest, as well as how and when to emerge from rest.

3.5 Applying the Goldilocks Principle to New and Newish Concussions

Finding the Goldilocks point—not too much, not too little activity—is very useful for your recovery.

3.6 Symptom-Action Frameworks

To help you get the right activity-to-rest balance, I provide you with two different symptom-action frameworks. One symptom-action framework is appropriate for up to three months from your concussion event, the other for more than three months (i.e., Persistent Post-Concussive Symptoms).

3.7 In Recovering from PPCS, How Hard and Fast Should I Push Myself?

This a challenging question, and at this point, there is no definite answer. In this section, I explain some possible answers, and, subsequently, my approach for how to more comfortably return a PPCS patient to their activities.

3.8 Fatigue

Arguably, fatigue is one of the most debilitating of PPCS symptoms. To better understand your fatigue, I give you an analogy I call "your summer versus your winter brain."

> ### 3.9 A DIY Approach to Relieving Fatigue
> There are a number of effective drugless treatments that you can undertake yourself. These will not only help you with your fatigue but greatly speed up the process of getting back to normal.
>
> ### 3.10 When Not to Go It Alone
> I review a number of reasons you may want to seek professional help instead of going it alone.

3.1 How Zara Overcame Fatigue

On a sunny weekend morning, Zara was riding her bike to meet a friend for brunch. After a long, dark winter, she was looking forward to being able to sit out on a patio for the first time. While crossing an intersection, her front wheel got jammed in a streetcar track, throwing her forcefully to the ground. Fortunately, her helmet took the brunt of the impact. She was quickly able to get up and orient her bike. But then she needed to sit for a while. Almost immediately, she developed a headache and neck pain.

That Monday, she consulted her family doctor, who diagnosed a concussion. The only indication she might have a longer recovery was a history of ADHD that had been diagnosed in her teens. Her doctor gave her advice on the use of over-the-counter headache medications and referred her to an occupational therapist (OT) and physiotherapist (PT) team. Due to her financial limitations, Zara was not able to consult this team for more than four or five sessions. During her first session, her OT gave Zara some important self-management tools for pacing, planning, and sleep hygiene. On the second week, her PT carried out a graduated concussion cardio stress test. Based on the results of this test, the PT prescribed a progressive home-based cardio program. The PT then focused on her headaches and neck pain. It turned out that these were quickly alleviated by a small number of in-clinic, hands-on therapy sessions, along with a home program of stretches and strengthening exercises (see chapter 5).

Later in her recovery, Zara's OT gave her a work-conditioning program at a local library (see chapter 8). This enabled Zara to return to her clerical work in three months. Her fatigue still persisted, albeit to a much lesser degree. At this point, she described her fatigue as being more mental than physical. By the end of the week, she would feel mentally drained. It would take her a whole weekend of little activity to be ready to start the cycle over again the next week. Frustrated, she felt she was stuck at about 75 percent of her full stamina.

Her doctor referred her to a neurologist, who recommended a trial of methylphenidate (e.g., Ritalin). This helped her overcome the last barrier to returning to her former self. All told, to fully recover, it took Zara six months of her own efforts, combined with selective sessions with four different clinicians.

3.2 Energy, the Final Frontier

When it comes to recovering from a concussion, metabolic energy (not the New Age, woo-woo crystal type of energy!) is the final frontier. This is also true, but to a lesser degree, for Persistent Post-Concussive

Symptoms (PPCS). For those with concussion/PPCS, by the evening, your symptoms will generally be greater and your ability to do almost anything less.

Why is this? Your brain needs extra energy for healing. However, because the brain is *potentially* inflamed, its ability to give itself sufficient energy, even for regular day-to-day activities, drops. The result is an energy crisis within the brain (see Section 3.3 "Deep Dive: The Concussed Brain's Energy Crisis"). This energy gap is felt, especially by the newly concussed, as fatigue. Unfortunately, why this tendency to fatigue persists for PPCS is very poorly understood.

Here are three analogies to help you to better visualize and manage your energy. Keep in mind that analogies are always simplifications of quite complex issues. Nevertheless, they will give you useful images to latch on to and to use in your day-to-day tasks.

Your Brain's Empty Gas Tank

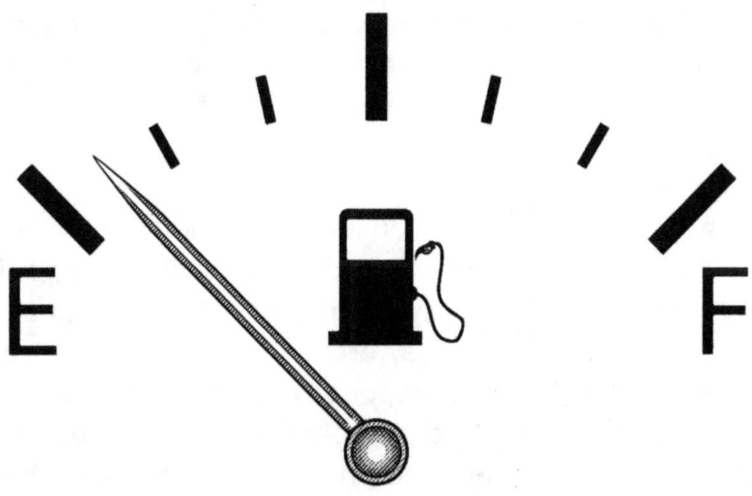

Your brain's energy stores can be compared to the tank of a car. When you have gas, you can run along just fine. But when you don't, you will have more difficulty doing even the simplest of things and have many more symptoms, including fatigue.

Taking this analogy a bit further, not only is your gas tank much smaller than normal, you also have less capacity to refill it. All told, this means you run out of energy much faster than before, and once your tank is empty, it takes you much more time to rebuild your resources.

Your Energizer Bunny Brain
The gas tank analogy is quite good, but when a car runs out of gas, it stops. You don't. Like the very popular "Energizer Bunny," you just keep on going. You can draw on energy from tomorrow's pool to do what you "need" to do today. The trouble is, when tomorrow comes, you find you're already out of juice. My patients find this analogy very helpful in understanding their delayed symptom onset, as well as the boom-and-bust economy of their energy levels. Early concussion patients often report the following experience: one day they are doing just fine, and the next they are so "symptom-y" and fatigued that the day is a virtual write-off.

Your Brain's Batteries
Another helpful analogy comes from Clark Elliot's book *The Ghost in My Brain*.[1] Being a professor of artificial intelligence, he naturally thinks in terms of images involving electrical circuits, etcetera. Based on his very long PPCS recovery, he proposed that the brain's energy reserve is best thought of as being like three batteries in a series. Metaphorically, he proposes, we all have these batteries.

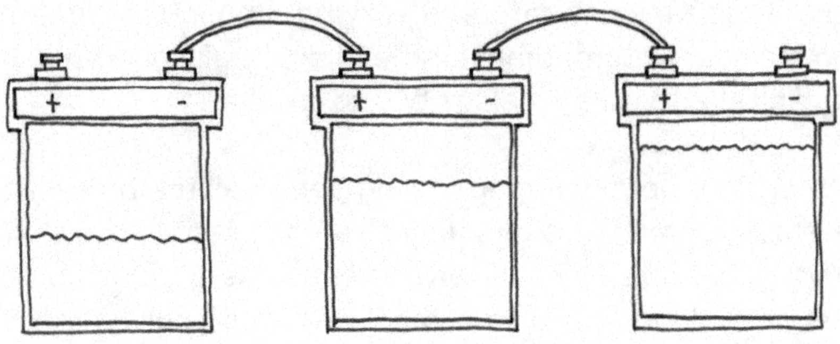

The first battery is your short-term battery, one that continually goes up and down during the day. You finish a tiring task and feel pooped. You sit down for a bit then, in relatively short order, you're ready to go again. The next battery in the series is a medium-term one. It takes more time to discharge and recharge. For example, you have worked all week and you need the weekend to revive.

The final battery is a long-term battery. This one is used less often and takes a lot to discharge. As an example, Professor Elliot uses the situation where your child is in the hospital. By the time you have been up for seventy-two hours straight, you're totally exhausted. Once it's all over, it will likely take you a couple of weeks to bounce back.

He believes that concussed/PPCS individuals go through their energy reserves much more quickly than the average person. In addition, they use higher levels of batteries much sooner than they would normally. Finally, he proposes that a person can't charge a given battery until the proceeding battery is fully charged up. This is a helpful way of thinking about the situation, because it explains why concussed individuals, depending on how and what they do, can take varying amounts of time to bounce back. Sometimes, if they have really overdone it, it can take them a week or two to recover.

Other than not ending up feeling poorly all the time, why is staying on an energy budget so important in the short and medium term? Your brain needs energy, not just to get stuff done, but also to heal. So if all your energy is going to your children, spouse, friends, and employer, then very little is going to you and your healing!

One final point: too little activity will slow your recovery just as too much will, maybe even more. If you continually overdo or underdo it, your condition *may* become chronic (i.e., Persistent Post-Concussive Symptoms—PPCS). I emphasize "may" because, as with many things, our understanding of why some individuals go on to PPCS is limited. One hypothesis is that going "chronic" is due to a poor rest /activity balance.

3.3 Deep Dive: The Concussed Brain's Energy Crisis

<u>Concussion</u>

How a concussion works deep down (aka its pathophysiology) is a very complex subject, far too complex for this book. Nevertheless, it is worthwhile to understand it in very broad strokes, as it explains the reasons for your fatigue. It is not just in your head. It is, but ... well, you get the picture.

Your neurons, the tiny workhorses of your thinking, have a complex energy cycle (aka metabolism).

Neurons that have been impacted by a concussion event can't "eat" and get the energy they need to do their work properly. Think how you would feel, and how little you could accomplish, if you hadn't eaten for a long while. How does this happen? As discussed in chapter 1, concussion events lead to movements that can *potentially* cause injury to neurons and/or their connections. If this cellular damage happens, it does so seemingly randomly, right across the brain. Animal experiments show that such damage causes an unusual and unwelcome release of ions and neurotransmitters, the chemical communicators of your brain. This stops the neurons from being able to operate in their normal electrical fashion. [2]

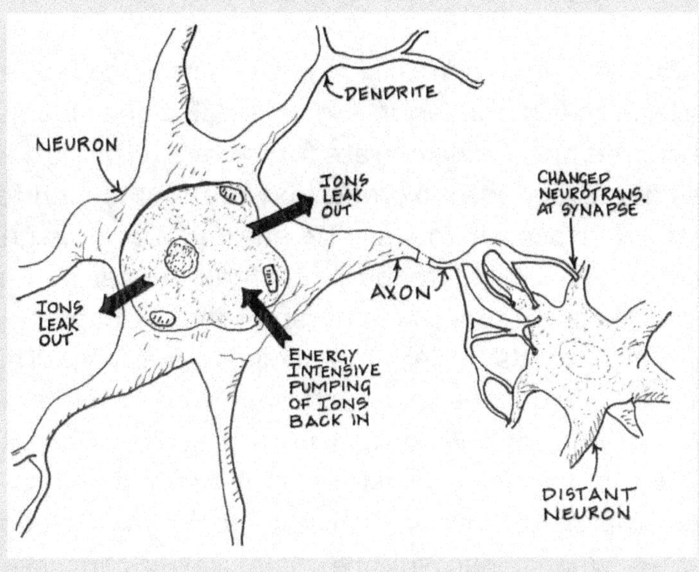

Your neurons really don't like this situation and will work very, very hard, consuming a large amount of their energy in the process, to try to pump out unwanted ions and rebalance their neurotransmitters (to restore homeostasis). But this increased energy has to come from somewhere. In the brain, ultimately, that energy comes from glucose. In both the body and the brain, glucose is in turn converted into adenosine triphosphate (ATP).[2] You can think of ATP as a kind of energy currency, or the way your brain pays to get its work done. Another way of thinking about it is like burning wood to heat a house. The brain "burns" ATP to release the energy stored in it. In addition, the brain's ability to use its own energy sources relies on having enough oxygen in your blood and getting rid of the "carbon dioxide by-product" of burning the ADP.

Unfortunately, a concussion is also known to lead to a decrease in the brain's own local blood supply. While the brain is desperate for more energy, it now has decreased local oxygen, oxygen that is vital for it to gain access to its ATP energy. Less oxygen means less ability to burn its fuel. In very short order, a newly concussed person runs out of energy, entering what's called metabolic depression. This causes a widespread reduction in what your brain can do, and for how long. A perfect storm of events results in an energy crisis in your brain. There is a real mismatch between what your brain needs versus what it can supply itself. Newly concussed individuals, then, experience profound fatigue, poor mental endurance, and the need to sleep a lot. [2]

<u>Persistent Post-Concussive Symptoms</u> (PPCS)

What about PPCS? Why does this low energy and fatigue persist to a degree long after the concussion, or inflammation, is thought to be over? Recent research suggests that it isn't the result of just one thing. Instead, PPCS is very likely from multiple and often overlapping issues. At the cellular level, it's thought to result from ongoing problems with your local blood supply: the delivery of oxygen and the elimination of carbon dioxide and other metabolic by-products. It might also relate to damage of the nerves connecting your neurons, the white matter of the brain. Some suggest it is due to underdiagnosed neck issues (see chapters 5 and 6). Others propose underdiagnosed or untreated sleep problems (see chapter 4). Finally, there are all the important, and just as real, psychological contributions: stress, mood/anxiety, and your coping skills.

Who's on first when it comes to long-term fatigue? We don't really know, but it's most likely for reasons unique to the individual. Your lack of energy is indeed in your head, but not, as some around you might imply, just in your imagination!

3.4 To Rest or Not to Rest, That Is the Question

In the early days of a concussion, your doctor may have told you to rest, but you do not know what that means, nor how long to stay there, nor how to come out of rest. The *2023 Consensus Statement on Concussion in Sport* recommended that such total physical and cognitive rest, if needed at all, should be limited to no more than twenty-four to forty-eight hours.[3] Thereafter, it's important for both the quality and speed of recovery that concussed individuals should gradually, as tolerated, become active (e.g., walking or stationary bike). They should do this while avoiding risky activities that could involve contact, collision, or the risk of falling.

<u>Early On, What Is and Isn't Rest</u>?
This is not as easy to define as you might think. What you thought of as restful before, like getting together with some friends for lunch, is no longer restful for you post a concussion. In the early days of a concussion, it's easier in many ways to define what is not restful or needs to be limited. This includes:
- being under bright, especially flickering, lights;
- exposure to loud environments/clanging sounds;
- strenuous and/or prolonged activity;
- prolonged reading;
- gatherings or meetings (i.e., with more than two people); and
- screen time on desktops, especially scrolling on handheld devices and, to a lesser degree, TV.

Total avoidance of screens longer than forty-eight hours from the injury has not proven that effective. But use common sense. If your symptoms increase to more than two out of ten on a scale of ten (where ten is the worst you can imagine), back off. Similarly, if a lesser symptom load results but lasts for a longish period (i.e., sixty minutes), this is too much for you at that time. [3]

3.5 Applying the Goldilocks Principle to New and Newish Concussions

Most people remember from their childhood the story of "Goldilocks and the Three Bears." If not, it's about how a young girl named Goldilocks ate a bear's bowl of porridge which was "not too hot, not too cold, but just right." I'm using this story now to show how to achieve the right balance between activity and rest for concussions (this information doesn't apply to PPCS), especially earlier on in the condition.

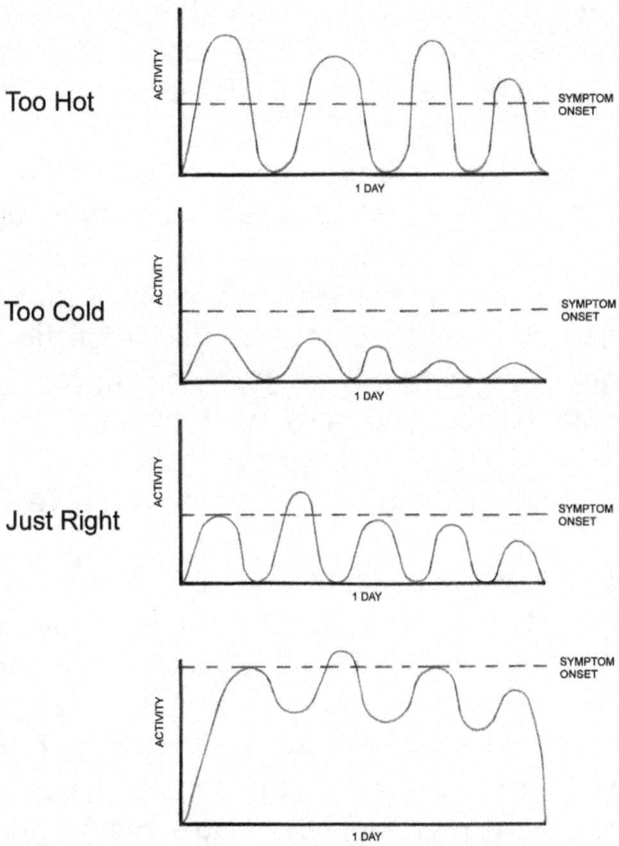

Graphs adapted from those used in the Regional Acquired Brain Injury Program, St Joseph's Health Care, London Ont.

The graphs above represent different approaches to activity levels and the onset of symptoms over a given day. The concussed individual usually starts the day with low or no symptoms. As they become more active, their symptoms tend to show or increase greatly. For all the graphs, the area below the dashed line represents when they have very low symptoms or are symptom-free. The top "too-hot graph" shows when an individual repetitively overdoes their activities.

Often, they ignore their increasing discomfort until their symptoms become so strong, they are forced back to rest. Over the day, they repeat this behaviour. Many individuals adopt this kind of boom-and-bust approach to activity when they are first concussed.

In contrast, the second "too-cold graph" shows an individual who is afraid of getting any symptoms and therefore does very little. In this case, the patient never challenges the brain to recover. Recovery via neuroplasticity (see chapter 2) is difficult for the brain. If it can get away with it, it will try to not have to do this. The problem is that you will stay in this very small world unless you challenge your brain to accommodate and recover. Doing nothing will not promote recovery!

The third "just-right graph" shows an individual who is trying to stay, more often than not, around their symptom threshold. They do this by appropriately budgeting their available energy (see below). Each time the patient's symptoms increase, they take a brief break (often five minutes is enough, see the mini meditation below) and resume activity, preferably by doing something different. If they are doing something mental, they switch over to something physical. Note that they do not need to be perfect and can occasionally overdo it. That's absolutely okay and is in no way damaging their brain.

The final graph shows what happens to the individual when they keep on budget, more often than not, around their symptom threshold. Gradually they can do more and more with less rest. But if the person mostly adopts either the too-hot or too-cold behaviour, they will prolong their recovery and *may* develop a more chronic condition. Later in this chapter, I will give you a number of tools to help you achieve this difficult balancing act.

3.6 Symptom-Action Frameworks

This is all well and good in theory. But how do you know when you are overdoing it? To help work this out, I will give you two symptom-action frameworks: one for the concussion period (except for the first two days when rest is advised), and the other for the Persistent Post-Concussive Symptoms period.

<u>Symptom-Action Framework Appropriate for the concussion period</u>
Use this from day three to one month form your injury date. [4]

Here are the four rules for you to follow during this period:
1. If you have a given symptom (a headache, say), be as active as you can, but try not to worsen the symptom. If a symptom increases more than a two out of ten (where ten is the worst you can imagine for that symptom), STOP, take five minutes' rest (e.g., mini meditation, see below), then switch to doing

something different. If you were doing something mental (e.g., doing insurance paperwork—egad), switch to doing something physical (e.g., go for a walk—phew!).

2. If a new symptom appears, STOP and take five minutes' rest. Then switch to doing something different as above.

3. Pay attention to your symptoms the next day. If you wake up with stronger symptoms compared to the end of the day before, this does not mean you have done any one thing wrong. Instead, it means you have overdone it with your total previous day's activities.

4. While doing specific exercises, your symptoms may increase. This is okay so long as the increase is tolerable for you, and so long as your symptoms return to their pre-exercise level within about sixty minutes.[2] If not, you will need to decrease the difficulty, repetitions, and/or duration of your exercises so you don't break this rule.

For a form you can copy, see Appendix C and
https://www.paulgodlewski.com/concussion-exercise-tools-
and-appendices/

If you can't always follow these guidelines, *don't worry: you are not causing yourself harm.* You are not going to be perfect at this, but again, that's fine. These rules are just recommendations to speed up your recovery, and are more important the newer your concussion is.

<u>Symptom-Action Framework Appropriate for the PPCS period</u> (i.e., beyond one month)
The following symptom-action framework was designed for the older term PCS (i.e., starting at three-month mark from the injury). It came from a conference presentation made by neurologist Dr. Jeffrey Kutcher.[5] From his talk, he

recommends four different rules for PCS. Based on the PPCS approach, I start applying this framework earlier on (i.e., from the one-month mark onwards).

- If you are experiencing annoying symptoms, your approach is to ignore them.
- If you are experiencing aggravating symptoms, in other words, worse than just annoying but still tolerable, your approach is to try to put up with them.
- If your symptoms become intolerable, you need to change your activities (in degree and/or duration), so that your symptoms are merely annoying or aggravating the next time around. To Dr Kutcher's third rule I add: it's best that you also modulate your activity level so that any symptom that arises on any given day, even if tolerable, doesn't persist into the next day.
- Avoidance is not the best policy at this stage. Moderating your activities is a better approach.

For a form you can copy, see Appendix C or https://www.paulgodlewski.com/concussion-exercise-tools-and-appendices/

3.7 In Recovering from PPCS, How Hard and Fast Should I Push Myself?

These are challenging questions that even very experienced clinicians struggle with. This is because we don't have the research to guide us. It therefore comes down to clinical reasoning and one's experience as a clinician. Clinical experience really amounts to what your patients have taught you (or tried to teach you) over the years. So, let's begin there with three stories, two from my own patients and another from Sarah Polley's book, *Run Towards the Danger*. [6]

A couple of years ago, I had a PCS patient (i.e., one having symptoms and functional limitations greater than three months post injury). She had finally managed to return to her challenging management work. She was coping very well, but by the end of each work week she was very fatigued. This went on for a while, so much so that she referred to this phenomenon as her "glass ceiling." She just couldn't seem to get past this limitation in her energy level.

At one point, her work required her to attend a weeklong work retreat. Generally, work retreats are anything but a retreat. She dreaded the idea of the near-constant meetings this entailed, some of which she attended. This, combined with air travel, sleeping in a strange room, and eating unhealthy food, seemed the perfect pathway to exhaustion.

She was delighted and exhilarated to get to the end of the week and discover she had coped very well. Unfortunately, that weekend she crashed with a two- to three-day-long headache and profound fatigue. It was not until Tuesday of the following week that she was able to go back to work. Even then, she was still quite tired. The odd thing was, and very surprising to both of us, she discovered thereafter that her glass ceiling was gone.

Here's another story, this time about a registered massage therapist with PCS. Over many months, he had consulted me from time to time. While he improved for a while, he plateaued at one point and was still unable to return to his work. Given our lack of progress, I discharged him back to his doctor's care and, to break the logjam, I recommended some alternate treatment approaches he might want to try.

Some months later, he contacted me to tell me that he was back to his work full-time and with full duties. A month after stopping treatments with me (being then more than one year since the injury), his insurance company declined to cover any further treatments and cut off his income coverage. As his family could not afford having no income from him, he felt obligated to go back to work. He reported that the initial eight to ten weeks back were "brutal." But having weathered this, he then strangely started to feel increasingly better. In the end, he felt he had fully recovered his former self.

The final story is from the book written by the director and actor Sarah Polley.[6] To avoid spoiling too much of her book, I'll just relate that she was finally able to beat her prolonged PPCS only by aggressively challenging herself. Her initial assessment and program were done in the US under experienced multidisciplinary medical care. In her case, she accomplished her goals with a mainly home-based program over an incredibly short six-week period. Her book is well worth a read for anyone struggling with chronic PPCS (i.e., more than six to twelve months post-injury). The approach that worked so well for her is most suited to PPCS, especially chronic forms of it, as in her case. It is *not* suitable for new or newish concussions.

How should we interpret these three stories? With some cautions (see following), these examples taught me that a PPCS patient's symptoms and limitations *may* be top-down imposed by the brain. But once these patients' particular "glass ceilings" were shattered, it forced their brains to reevaluate both the actual level of threat as well as their physical, cognitive, and emotional limitations. Finally, these stories indicate that recovery *can* be in the order of weeks rather than months.

Here are some cautions about this approach:

- Engaging and inspiring, these stories may hint at a greater truth, a new principle. But as clinicians, we need to be cautious about drawing general principals from such a low number of cases. Hopefully, research will address this problem soon.
- This kind of rapid and aggressive program requires the individual to be able to tolerate a fair amount of discomfort for a longish period. Some PPCS sufferers will not have the needed family support and personal resources to cope with this. For many, there is a slower, stepwise approach that can work just as well (see below).
- I would definitely not recommend "going it alone" in this kind of case. In fact, in chapters 8 and 9, which cover returning to activity, I recommend that it's always best to do this kind of thing under experienced medical supervision. Preferably, this care should be multidisciplinary and coordinated. In Sarah's case, she received care from an experienced US-based concussion team, Michael Collins, Phd (Clinical and Neuropsychology), and physiotherapist Anne Mucha, DPT (Neurological & Vestibular PT). Such good clinicians are to be found both in Canada and the US.
- As stated above, this aggressive approach is not suitable for a person with an early concussion. When you should consider doing something like this is hotly debated. My rule of thumb is to gradually apply this strategy at the onset of the PPCS (i.e., one-plus months). By the three-month mark (i.e., the beginning of the older PCS model), with some exceptions, I am very comfortable being more aggressive with my exercise prescription and returning to activity recommendation.

- For some unlucky individuals, the ceiling is not glass at all, but concrete. This is because they potentially have more profound degrees and/or extents of injury. Repeatedly hammering away at it will not necessarily cause a breakthrough. In these cases, it leads to unrelenting, often escalating symptoms, with little in the way of functional gains.
- Every concussion and PPCS case is unique. They therefore need to be medically evaluated on that basis.

Before making my own recommendations for how a person with PPCS should ramp up their activities, I want to discuss the Twin Peaks Model of Pain.[7]

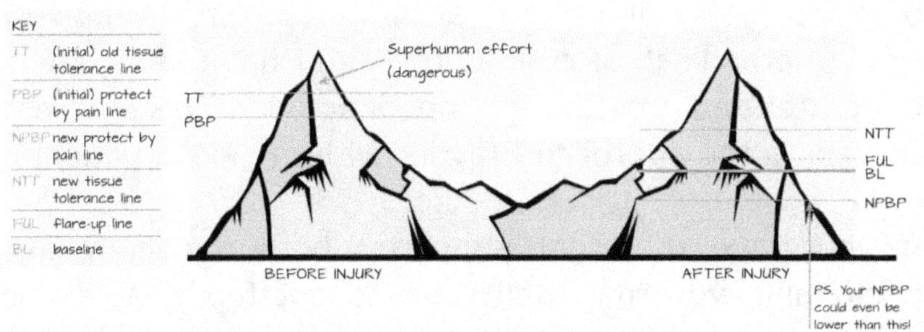

©2013 - Permission for use given by NOI Group. [7]
www.noigroup.com

This is a model for how many PTs deal with chronic pain. It is not directly applicable to PPCS, but I think we can still draw some lessons from it.

All tissues have tolerance for how much load they can take. This can be imagined as a mountain. Olympic athletes have to train long and hard to be nearer the top of this mountain. For most of us mere mortals, the tissue's tolerance is down the mountain. Your pain system is designed to alert you when you are starting to get close to your personal maximum. When someone has been injured—let's say a shoulder—the injured shoulder tissue's capacity to do its job is lessened. Once this happens, the pain system is automatically reset, but seemingly at a lower level to protect tissue and help it recover.

In this model of chronic pain, it's hypothesized that the pain system is kept artificially low because it has not been sufficiently challenged. This low level of pain tolerance gets entrenched, and the new low becomes the person's new norm for dealing with pain. Under this model, treatment for chronic pain sufferers involves re-educating their pain system to become less vigilant and reactive. Generally, this is accomplished in a relatively slow, methodical, step-like process of habituating them to greater and greater amounts of activity. This stepwise process is the approach I favour with my PPCS patients.

If you have the right supports, both medically and personally, you may well want to opt for a rapid and aggressive program. Moreover, it may be necessary if someone has very chronic PPCS, like Sarah Polley's (three and a half years!). However, there is no evidence to say that it has to be done this way.

As a clinician, when I am given the opportunity, I like to begin much earlier and stepwise to increase my PPCS patient's activity tolerance, neither being too timid nor too aggressive with them. I think this is a more comfortable way for them to recover their world. The downside is that it does take more time. In addition, my suspicion is that it needs to be done as early in the PPCS recovery process as possible (i.e., my preference at the three-plus months' mark).

3.8 Fatigue

Early on after a concussion, and for a time following the event, fatigue is entirely normal. However, fatigue often continues into PPCS and is arguably one of its most debilitating symptoms. Our understanding of Persistent Post-Concussive Symptoms fatigue is, unfortunately, still very much in its infancy. The first task is for you to check with your doctor so they can rule out issues such as: deficiencies in your iron, vitamin B12, blood sugar problems, etcetera.

Beyond these things, which are simple to check, many overlapping factors are often at the root of a concussed person's fatigue. These include, but are not limited to:
- the increased mental effort of doing even very basic tasks;
- sleep disturbance, also sometimes associated with concussion and PPCS; and
- mood disturbances.

An analogy I came up with—*"your summer brain versus your winter brain"*—will give you sense of why you have fatigue. Your brain has a preferred and most efficient processing speed. Despite having a concussion/PPCS, your brain will do its best to return to this speed, somewhat independent of your new capacity.

Prior to the injury, your brain was like a car just gliding along a summer road at 120 km/hr (75 mph). The concussed brain will continue to try to drive as quickly as it can, but now it's having to do this on a windy, icy road, plowing all the while through the snow. For every kilometer of road (i.e., every quantum of thinking), the winter brain has to work so much harder compared to the summer brain. This helps to explain the sunset effect, and why a concussed person is "toast" by the end of the day or after a bout of hard thinking. Many things that were formerly a snap, like chatting with a group of friends, will suck the very gas right out of you. Even basic social activities take a surprising amount of mental processing, energy now in very short supply. In virtually no time at all, group interactions will drain the concussed/PPCS patient dry.

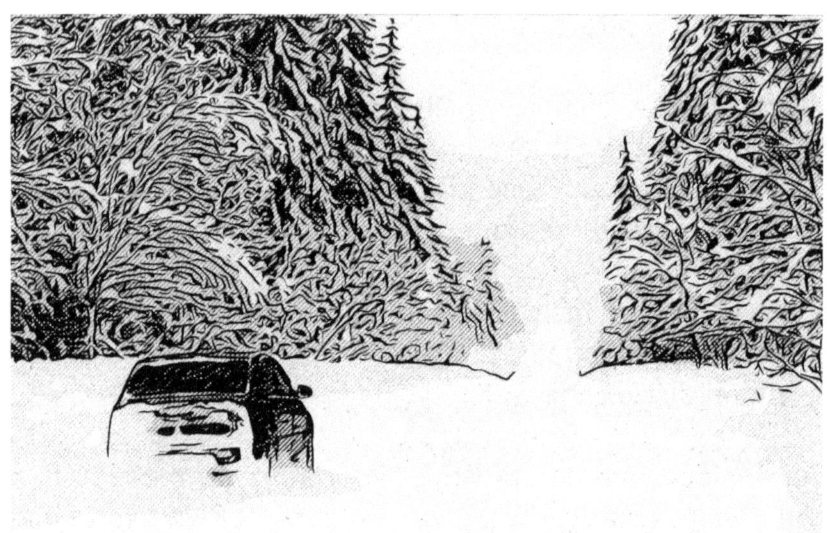

3.9 A DIY Approach to Relieving Fatigue

All the tools that follow are helpful. But they are particularly beneficial when used in combination.

<u>A Mini-Meditation to Relax and Reboot the Brain</u>
When neurons in the brain are injured, they don't go quiet but become noisy, producing random signals. The concussed brain is like a radio station that has been bumped off its signal/station. As a result, the radio-brain

is full of static. Quieting via meditation allows the brain to better perceive that it's off-signal and learn to get back onto station. This mini-meditation helps to quieten the brain and to replenish its depleted energy reserves. Taking a break from thoughts and feelings, even if briefly, will also give your brain a break from your worries and ruminations.

Do this mini-meditation any time you feel your symptoms begin to rise. This is particularly helpful at the beginning of a concussion (aka an acute concussion), when the brain feels especially threatened and is in fight-or-flight crisis. As such, the brain can become overly excited and watchful for possible future threats.

When you are first learning mini-meditation, sit comfortably in a dark and quiet room. Don't lie down as you will likely fall asleep. Put a timer on to avoid napping while meditating. Breathe slowly and rhythmically (approximately twelve breaths per minute, but don't count them; just slow them to what is comfortable for you). Breathe in through the nose, out through your mouth. You don't need to push the air out; just relax and let the air pass out of your open mouth. Breathe deeply enough so that the air you take in expands both your upper and lower chest and swells your tummy a bit. This type of breathing causes a relaxation response in the whole body, including the brain.

While deep breathing, an added practice to help calm the visual system is to use one of two additional techniques:
- For part of the time, try to visualize the colour called midnight black (i.e., black velvet, dipped in water). By doing this, you are "tricking" your visual system to quieten down even more. This will cause you to relax

further, especially around the eyes, which in turn reduces headaches and discomfort.

- Alternatively, for those who have difficulty visualizing, you can do a mindfulness technique. As you breathe in, feel the cool air going down your throat and into your lungs. As you breathe out, concentrate on the mottled black at the back of your eyelids.

Both these visualization techniques can be helpful but are not as important to the relaxation process as the deep, slow rhythmical breathing. If you can't do either, don't sweat it.

A brief word about being distracted by stray thoughts while meditating. This is inevitable and doesn't mean you're a *"bad meditator."* Note for you type As (including myself), being a good meditator is not the object of this exercise. Its purpose is to relax the brain.

Think of the stray thoughts as trains coming into a station. The doors of this train open up, inviting you to "come onboard." Try if you can to avoid getting onto that train of thought. Inevitably, however, you will find yourself off in la-la land. Do not get all stressed about this. Simply note it, get off the train, and resume your deep breathing, plus or minus one of the visualizations. It's more important to get off the train frequently than to try to stop getting on the trains of thought (not very relaxing).

Meditate frequently, say six times per day, for five minutes. (It is not important that you do it exactly six times per day. Just do it as frequently as your symptoms present themselves.)

At first, you only really need to do this in a quiet, dark room. Once you've learned the technique, you can and should do it almost anywhere. Find a comfortable quiet place to sit, lean forward, and cup your eyes with your hands to block out most of the light. If you have earplugs, use those too to reduce the sound stimulation coming into your brain. Having initially trained yourself to do this in a quiet room, your brain will recognize it ("*Oh, this!*") and begin to relax.

Please note, meditation works for most people, but it is not for everyone. Stop if you start to become overly anxious or depressed while, or after, meditating. For some people, a mindfulness walk works better (see chapter 6).

<u>Pacing and Planning</u>
It's very important, especially in the early days of a concussion, to both pace out and plan for activities. Pacing and planning (P&P) are two simple words that are remarkably hard to put into effect in anyone's life!

Below, I provide you with three tools to help you P&P. Bear in mind that these are just tools. I once knew a doctor who was fond of saying: "If the cure is worse than the disease, chuck it!" Similarly, if any of these tools is not helpful, too onerous, unduly stresses you out, or makes your symptoms worse, chuck it! Also, feel free to simplify or adapt it to what works best for you.

- A timer for pacing and planning. Especially in the early days, a simple timer can come in handy for P&P. These days, all mobile phones have one. If you don't have a mobile, use a digital watch timer or an egg timer. Set the timer to remind you to take a break and move on to something different. This will stop you from becoming absorbed in a given task at the expense of your symptoms and the other things you need to accomplish. Taking insufficient breaks will cause your symptoms to spike, and you will feel more tired the next day.[4]

- Activity Versus Symptom Journal (Plus or Minus Mood). A journal that charts your activities versus your symptoms can be very helpful in the early days of a concussion. Concussions and PPCS are always evolving. Like a snapshot, the journal will teach you about your concussion at given times. It's also useful later on when you're making a big change in your routine (e.g., going back to work). Concussions are like snowflakes; they are all different. Teaching yourself about *your* concussion at this moment is important. If you are unfortunate enough to have another one, it would again be important for you to learn about that one too. [4]

Activity versus Symptom Journal (+/- Mood)

	Morning				Afternoon				Evening			
	Symptom	/ 10 Mood	LM	A	Symptom	/ 10 Mood	LM	A	Symptom	/ 10 Mood	LM	A
Day 1												
	Symptom	/ 10 Mood	LM	A	Symptom	/ 10 Mood	LM	A	Symptom	/ 10 Mood	LM	A
Day 2												

For a form you can copy, see Appendix D or
https://www.paulgodlewski.com/concussion-exercise-tools-and-appendices/

Three times a day (e.g., after breakfast, after lunch, and at bedtime), globally rate all your concussion symptoms on a scale of one to ten, where ten is the worst you can imagine. You shouldn't itemize each type of symptom, just as an overall symptom score for that portion of the day. In addition, by circling it, you may want to note how your mood is: low mood (LM) and/or anxious (A). It's not always obvious what's emotionally impacting you. Adding this information can give you clues as to what is consistently lowering your mood and/or making you anxious. If you're consulting a psychological counsellor, they will find this information quite helpful.

The journal has seven rows, each for a different day of a given week. You can do more if you find it very helpful. But one week is usually sufficient. Break up your day into morning, afternoon, and evening. For each portion of your day, note your activities in point form. You don't need to go into a lot of detail. Just include a bit about the following: the task itself, the environment in which you did it, and roughly how long it took (e.g., *two friends, busy/noisy café, 30 mins.*).

Most often, you'll note there's not a big connection between your activity at one time and your symptoms soon thereafter. By the end of the day (aka the sunset effect), your symptoms will start to correlate to that day's activity level. Often, the number and degree of symptoms (e.g., high fatigue) will only show up the next morning. Pay attention to both. They don't indicate you did anything wrong and, more importantly, you did not do your brain any harm. They just indicate that your density of activity was too high for that day.

I am not a great believer in concussion symptom *"triggers."* Often, concussed individuals will note that they can do the same activity and have radically different symptom levels. This is because your level of symptoms is more related to your energy state at the time. I subscribe to the notion that certain activities are *"gas guzzlers"* of your energy rather than symptom *"triggers."*

The purpose of the journal is for you to learn not only your limits but also which activities you tolerate well and even make you feel better. So, don't be afraid to play and experiment with your activities. Apart from risky behaviours you need to avoid, such as jarring yourself or falling, you won't make your concussion worse. *Hurt does not equal harm.* You are simply teaching yourself how to P&P in order to stay within your available energy budget.

- The week ahead planning tool
  I have found the following tool most useful for those of my patients trying to significantly increase their activity, such as getting back to work. But it can be used at any time during the recovery process. [4]

Appendix F
Week ahead planning tool

Use to plan what optimally you would like to do. Start by filling in what you do regularly (e.g., getup, breakfast, etc.). Then things you regularly have to do (e.g., children pickup, work, etc.). Then add exercise & R&R times.

	MON	TUES	WED	THURS	FRID	SAT	SUN
06:00 - 06:30							
06:30 - 07:00							
07:00 - 07:30							
07:30 - 08:00							
08:00 - 08:30							
08:30 - 09:00							
09:00 - 09:30							
09:30 - 10:00							
10:00 - 10:30							
10:30 - 11:00							

For a form you can copy, see Appendix E or
https://www.paulgodlewski.com/concussion-exercise-tools-
and-appendices/

Use the agenda for what you plan to do, not what you did in a given day. Like all planning exercises, they rarely work out just as you plan. Still, planning is a very worthwhile exercise because it will tell you what you are trying to accomplish. Regularly, failure is a sign that you need to adjust your expectations for a given day.

Start by allocating all the standard routines of the day: wake-up time, meals, and wind-down time before sleep. Next, put in all the things that you have to do—picking up your child at school, for example. Next, build in regular meditation breaks. Then add in time for the exercises outlined in this book. Don't worry about filling every available part of the day. It will be occupied by some unanticipated thing.

Before we finish talking about P&P, a quick note about the importance of being in control of your own activity level as much as possible. Let's say you want to meet a friend, or friends, at a café. Even though interacting with two friends will consume more of your energy, it is actually better for you to meet two friends than one. This is because you have more control and can leave more easily when it becomes too much for you. If it is just one person, you will feel socially obligated to stay past the point that is good for you. With two friends, you can say something like, "Guys, love you, but that's it for me. Perhaps next time I can stay for a bit longer." Hey, you touched base, reduced your chances of depression from isolation, and didn't expend too much energy. What's not to like about that?

In the second example, you want to go to a gathering at a friend's house. As in the first example, you need to find ways around the isolation that comes with concussions. Call your host/hostess in advance, explain the situation (don't hide your condition, as it causes no end of problems), and ask if there is a timeout space for you. Stay as long as you want, with a number of breaks. This way, you hit the sweet spot of going out but not overdoing it.

A Concussion Cardio Program to Rebuild Your Energy Budget

No one wants to live with such a small gas tank. This specialized brain cardio program will help restore your reserves. The downside of a regular cardiovascular workout, or worse, a "bootcamp" cardio program, is that it will increase blood pressure. With concussion, increased blood pressure often leads to increased symptoms, particularly headaches. By building in distinct steps, this concussion-tailored cardiovascular program helps to gradually habituate the brain to the higher blood pressures necessary for a normal life.

This concussion-tailored cardiovascular program is based on the work of Prof. John Leddy and colleagues at the University at Buffalo. Dr. Leddy and colleagues have found it safe to test patients with the Buffalo Concussion Treadmill Test (BCTT) as soon as two to ten days after the concussion event. [8] The reasons for doing this concussion-tailored cardiovascular program are much more complex than just energy restoration and involve overcoming concussion-related autonomic nervous system problems in the body. In addition, as we saw in chapter 2, it also leads to healing via promotion of good neuroplasticity.[8] But for this book's purposes, simplifying it under rebuilding energy capacity and reducing fatigue makes sense.

The research that Dr. Leddy's group carried out has been foundational to helping clinicians know what is safe and effective in the treatment of concussions and PPCS. To distinguish my approach from Dr. Leddy's, I call my program a modified, self-directed, concussion cardio (MSCC) program. This MSCC program is appropriate for those thirteen to sixty years of age. For safety reasons, this protocol is, by design, conservative. For example, I recommend my patients start no sooner than ten days from their concussion event. On a given day before they start, I also prefer that their overall symptoms to be no greater than a four or five out of ten, that their symptoms increase no more than two out of ten (where ten is the worst you can imagine) and persist no longer than sixty minutes after finishing exercising,[3] If any of this happens the patient needs to decrease how hard they are working and/or the length of their exercises. When trying this program, you should follow the same guidelines.

Remember, safety first: before starting this program, check with your family doctor if there is any reason you should not be doing this kind of workout. These include, but are not limited to:
- heart issues;
- increased risk for stroke;
- other vascular issues;
- lung issues;
- high blood pressure;
- electrolyte imbalance;
- mental or physical impairment leading to inability to exercise;
- medication issues; and
- musculoskeletal injuries.

If at any time while doing this cardio program you develop

shortness of breath or get dizzy, **STOP!** Consult your doctor. If you experience an irregular heartbeat or chest/arm/jaw/abdominal pain, call for an ambulance.

The equipment needed:
- Comfortable clothing for exercising (e.g., shorts, T-shirt, and running shoes)
- Water bottle
- Heart rate monitor (wrist style or chest strap monitors)
- Eventually, regular access to a stationary bike

Initially, I advise patients to walk outside (weather permitting) four times per week. I like my patients to walk every day. But I get them to alternate between this cardio walk and a mindful walk for sensory integration (see chapter 6). They need to warm up by walking quickly enough for two to five minutes to bring themselves to about 65 percent of their age-related target heart rate. The age-related heart rate maximum is calculated with a very simple formula: you simply subtract your age from 220. I recommend they start by walking for ten minutes, then cool down by walking more slowly for two to five minutes before stopping. Over the next two weeks, they increase the length of time they stay at the target heart rate by ten minutes. Once this is accomplished, they increase their target heart rate by five beats per minute (bpm) /week, as tolerated, but to no more than 85 percent of their age-related heart rate maximum.

Two examples will help flesh out how to apply all the numbers and establish your own program.
- Let's start with someone at the youngest age I would treat this way (twelve years of age). For a twelve-

year-old, the recommended maximum heart rate is 220 - 12 = 208 bpm. Sixty-five percent of this heart rate max would be 208 x 0.65 = 135 bpm. Their initial target heart rate range is 130-135 (rounding down). This would include a warmup of two to five minutes to 130-135 bpm, staying at this rate, on average, for ten minutes, and then cooling down for two to five minutes before stopping. They should walk a minimum of four times per week. Over the next two weeks, they should gradually increase their time at the target heart rate from a total of ten minutes to twenty minutes. Thereafter, as tolerated, they should increase their target heart rate by 5 bpm, but not exceed 177 bpm (i.e. (220 - 12) x 0.85).

- At the other end of the age spectrum, a sixty-year-old's recommended maximum heart rate is 220 - 60 = 160 bpm. Sixty-five percent of this heart rate max would be 220 x 0.65 = 104 bpm. Their initial target heart rate range is 100-105 (rounding up). This would include a warmup of two to five minutes to 100-105 bpm, staying on average at this rate for ten minutes, then cooling down for two to five minutes before stopping. They should walk a minimum of four times per week. Over the next two weeks, they should increase their time at the target heart rate from a total of ten minutes to twenty minutes. Thereafter, as tolerated, they should increase their target heart rate by 5 bpm, but not exceed 128 bpm (i.e. (220 - 60) x 0.85).

I recommend that those older than sixty consult their cardiologist, GP, or an experienced PT to establish their initial heart rate. There are often other issues (e.g., back, hip, and knee issues) which need to be taken into account when setting this level. For those under twelve, it is best to consult a pediatrician or a pediatric PT.

Walking outdoors has many benefits. But as the weeks go by, it will become increasingly difficult for the person to elevate their heart rate sufficiently just by walking faster. Initially, they can overcome this by incorporating hills and stairs into their program. But it's tricky to do this for a long period without getting a lot of spikes in heart rate and, therefore, blood pressure—something to be avoided, especially early on.

For this reason, I recommend the use of a simple stationary bike (either your own or at a fitness club). Access to a stationary bike is also useful for poor weather days or seasons. Treadmills are okay, but early on I recommend stationary bikes, as they are safer and produce fewer problems with dizziness for concussed individuals. I don't recommend ellipticals or StairMasters.

3.10 When Not to Go It Alone

There are a number of reasons why you may not want to go it alone. One is if you're daunted by the prospect of solitary exercise. The second is if you know in your heart of hearts that you're not likely to persist on your own. In both cases, depending on what the issue is, I recommend you consult the appropriate clinician who is experienced in dealing with concussions. For the issues covered in this chapter, you should seek a healthcare professional(s) if:

- With the passage of time, there has been little in the way of change in your fatigue. If it is lingering past approximately twelve to sixteen weeks, don't wait longer to seek help. Alternatively, if your fatigue is profound and unremitting, consult your GP and/or a neurologist. There are medications that can help.

- Despite the tools given above, you're finding it very difficult to prioritize, pace, and plan sufficiently. An occupational therapist is the best professional to consult.
- Prior to starting the cardio program, you have not met, or you are unsure if you have met, the safety criteria outlined above. Consult your doctor and/or a cardiologist.
- If, during the cardio program, you develop shortness of breath or get dizzy, ***STOP!*** Consult your doctor. If you experience an irregular heartbeat or chest/arm/jaw/abdominal pain, get someone to take you to the emergency department or call for an ambulance.

References

1. Elliot, Clark. 2015. *The Ghost in My Brain: How a Concussion Stole My Life and How the New Science of Brain Plasticity Helped Me Get It Back.* New York, USA Penguin.
2. Giza, Christopher presentation. 2016. "Mild Traumatic Brain Injury: Pathophysiology and Recovery." Traumatic Brain Injury Conference, University Health Network, Toronto, Canada.
3. Patricios J.S., et al. 2023. "Consensus Statement on Concussion in Sport: The 6th International Conference on Concussion in Sport–Amsterdam. October 2022." Br J Sports Med. 57, no. 11 (June), 695–711. https://doi.org/10.1136/bjsports-2023-106898
4. Modified from one used St Joseph's Hospital Acquired Brain Injury Program. Cited in McGuire, S. 2014 "Concussion Management Workshop." Bridgepoint Heath, Toronto, Ontario.
5. Kutcher, J.S. presentation. 2017. "Concussion and Long-Term Brain Health in Athletes." Traumatic Brain Injury Conference, University Health Network, Toronto, Canada.

6. Polley, Sarah. 2022. *Run Towards the Danger: Confrontations with a Body of Memory,* Toronto, Canada Hamish Hamilton a division of Penguin Random House.
7. Butler, D.S. and Mosle, G.L. 2013 *Explain Pain*, Noigroup Publication Adelaide, Australia.
8. Leddy J.J. et al. 2018. "Exercise is Medicine for Concussion." *Curr Sports Med Rep.* 17, no. 8 (Aug), 262-270. https://doi.org/10.1249/JSR.0000000000000505

Chapter 4

Problems with Sleep, Sensory Sensitivity, and Heightened Emotions

"Without enough sleep, we all become tall two-year-olds." JoJo Jensen

Cheat Sheet

4.1 How Tristan Overcame Sleep Disturbance, Sound Sensitivity and Anxiety

Tristan sustained a concussion from an assault. He struggled with sleep disturbance, sound sensitivity, and anxiety. Each was addressed by the right therapy at the right time.

4.2 Concussion's Early Days' Symptoms

Sleep disturbances, sensory sensitivities, and emotional distress are symptoms that show up early in the condition. I cover them all in this chapter as they are linked, both in terms of how they reinforce one another and how to treat them.

4.3 Sleep Disturbance

Sleep disturbance is very common, especially in the

early days of concussions. If needed, different types of treatment are often combined.

4.4 A DIY Approach to Relieving Sleep Disturbance

While there isn't much the patients themselves can do about physiological sleep problems that sometimes come with a concussion, they can do a lot to address the behavioural side of promoting good sleep.

4.5 Sound and/or Light Sensitivities

Fortunately, in the early days of a concussion, light and/or sound sensitivity usually go away by themselves. But for some individuals, these sensitivities can linger.

4.6 A DIY Approach to Relieving Sound and Light Sensitivities

The good news is that DIY treatments are quite effective. The basic principles for both of these sensory types are the same: understanding the sensitivity, time-limited use of such devices as sunglasses, earplugs, and graded exposure to the sound and/or light.

4.7 Emotional Issues Are No Less Real

Emotional issues play a big role in concussions and PPCS. Problems with emotional regulation may be an important consequence of concussion, and just as problematic as physical issues (e.g., a concussion-based headache).

> **4.8 When Not to Go It Alone**
> There are other reasons a concussed individual may not want to go it alone. For example, the prospect of doing exercises alone is daunting, or the sleep problems, sensitivities, and/or emotional issues are unremitting.

4.1 How Tristan Overcame Sleep Disturbance, Sound Sensitivity, and Anxiety

Coming home after a night out, Tristan and his partner were assaulted. Unfortunately, in trying to protect his partner, Tristan took the brunt of the attack. He very briefly lost consciousness. Coming to, he immediately experienced a strong headache, some tingling in his hands, and was very sensitive to both light and sound. None of the tests carried out at the local emergency department, including a CT scan, found any issues. The emergency physician diagnosed a concussion and discharged him to the care of his family doctor.

At home, Tristan started having issues with sleep, anxiety, and ringing in his ears (aka, tinnitus). Tristan had no prior problems with mood. His family doctor confirmed the diagnosis, recommended some medication, and referred him to an in-house occupational therapist (OT) well-experienced with treating concussions. His sleep was disturbed, but he reported he was not experiencing any nightmares or daytime flashbacks.

While his initial hand tingling and light sensitivity resolved quickly, he struggled with other ongoing symptoms. His sound sensitivity was high, and his tinnitus was quite loud at the end of the day or in certain situations. At times, he became quite irritable to the point of anger with sounds, particularly those generated by others. The OT worked with Tristan on the initial management of his mood issues, pacing, planning, sleep hygiene, and strategies to reduce sound sensitivity (see below).

Noting that they were not making much progress in helping him with his mood or reducing his sound sensitivity, his OT referred him to a registered clinical psychologist and to an audiologist, both knowledgeable in handling tinnitus and noise sensitivity. To help reduce the impact of tinnitus on Tristan's sleep, the audiologist recommended the nighttime use of a brown noise generator. She also recommended some specialized brain relaxation apps to help him with his tinnitus. The psychologist counselled Tristan using a combination of techniques, including Cognitive Behavioural Therapy (CBT) and graduated sound exposure and habituation exercises. All this gradually helped Tristan to reduce his sound sensitivity, irritability, and avoidance behaviours.

On the advice of the OT, Tristan's GP referred him to a sleep specialist. Through overnight and day studies, they found that, while he showed no issues with sleep apnea or restless legs, he had significant problems with getting to sleep for at least two hours per night. His sleep specialist therefore diagnosed Delayed Sleep-Wake (DSW) condition and prescribed melatonin, to be taken two hours before bed. This, and the sleep hygiene (see below), helped greatly to return his sleep to normal. All told, it took Tristin ten to twelve months to fully recover with the help of multiple practitioners handling different aspects of his care.

4.2 Concussion's Early Days' Symptoms

This chapter covers a number of issues, including sleep problems, sensory sensitivities, and emotional issues. I have chosen to address all these together because these symptoms appear early on and are often linked, reinforcing one another. After a concussion, and for a time following the event, having issues with your sleep, sound and/or light sensitivities, and being more emotional are all entirely normal. Thus, when experiencing such things, it's important to not worry.

4.3 Concussion-Related Sleep Disturbance

Following a concussion (mTBI), sleep disruption is very common. Up to 50 percent of TBI patients report sleep difficulties. About a third of these can be diagnosed with insomnia syndrome. This is approximately three times higher than for the regular population.[1] Counterintuitively, concussion patients are more likely than severe traumatic brain injury (TBI) patients to report such problems with their sleep.[2] If this is the case for you, it's best you discuss this with your GP and/or an experienced concussion clinician.

<u>Treatments for Concussion Sleep Disruption</u>
Treating sleep problems in individuals with concussion and PPCS is often more broad-based than targeted on one specific thing. For example, doctors may prescribe supplements (e.g., melatonin, zinc, or magnesium) before bedtime, along with sleep hygiene measure and body relaxation techniques.

4.4 A DIY Approach to Relieving Sleep Disturbance

I like to tell my patients that sleep is worth more than all the neurologists, physiotherapists (except maybe one, mentioning no names of course), occupational therapists, psychologists, psychological counsellors, and medication put together. Sleep is where the rubber hits the road for both healing and coping better with the day to come. A lot of neuroplastic changes and rewiring are thought to occur at night while sleeping. This is, after all, when you rebuild your energy reserves to meet the challenges of the next day.

While there isn't much the concussed person can do about physiological sleep problems that can come with concussion/PPCS, they do have a lot of control over the behavioural side of promoting good quality sleep.

Sleep quality trumps sleep quantity every time. It's far more important to get five hours of restorative sleep than ten hours of shallow sleep. But how do you know if you are getting good quality sleep? All things being equal (i.e., if you haven't overdone it the day before), if you feel neutral or more refreshed on awaking, then your sleep quality has been good.

<u>Sleep Hygiene</u> (Just who came up with that sexy name? How about Sensational Sleep?)
Sleep hygiene is the low-hanging fruit that should always be addressed before undergoing more formal sleep investigations and medications.

According to the Ontario Neurotrauma Guide, following a concussion you should try to start limiting your daytime naps after the first few days.[3] The thinking here is that napping will start to undermine nighttime sleep, making it harder to sleep through the night. As a rule of thumb, I recommend my patients sleep as much as they want during the night. Your system knows what it needs. So, give it free rein. The Ontario Neurotrauma Foundation recommends a number of additional things to promote good quality sleep for those with concussions: [3]

- Go to bed and wake up at the same time every day (an alternative approach is recommended below).
- After the first few days, avoid naps if you can. If you are very sleepy, try to take only one nap per day before 3:00 p.m., and keep it shorter than thirty minutes.
- Try to sleep in a bed. Don't fall asleep on the couch.
- Get some natural (outside) light during the day.
- Avoid heavy meals late in the evening.
- Consider having a bedtime snack that contains protein.
- Eat foods high in magnesium, iron, and B vitamins.
- Keep your bedroom free of electronic equipment such as computers, tablets, and cell phones. If this is not possible, turn them off or put them in "sleep" mode.
- Avoid using a digital clock with numbers that light up. If this cannot be avoided, turn it away from the bed and avoid looking at it during the night.

I learnt additional aspects of the behavioural side of sleep from Carney and Manber's book called *Goodnight Mind*.[4] It discusses how the sleep system works and how it can be modified, for good or ill, by your behaviours. Their approach differs a bit from the Ontario Neurotrauma Guide. The primary difference lies in their recommendations for waking and sleeping, as follows:[4]

- Sleep is aided by a cool, quiet bedroom. Other than sex, avoid doing anything stimulating like work or watching TV in bed. Sleep behaviour is very associative. Your body needs to associate the bedroom with sleep.
- Fix a regular wake-up time seven days a week.
- Allow your go-to-sleep time to initially float a bit, depending on how tired you are. Don't force yourself to go to bed. Don't try to fight with your sleep system. Rather, go to bed when you are feeling tired, even of this means you are going to bed later. Ah, but you still have to get up the next morning at your usual time—you'll likely drag yourself through the next day, and possibly be more symptomatic. But the next night, you'll probably sleep more deeply. By anchoring your wake-up period and allowing your bedtime to float, sleep time will seesaw, eventually setting itself to what you need.
- Exercising regularly, particularly in the afternoon, can help deepen sleep. However, avoid strenuous exercise two hours before bedtime.
- Generally, avoid alcohol. Avoid caffeine after noon (e.g., coffee, tea, many sodas, and chocolate) and spicy/sugary foods four to six hours before bed.
- For the two hours prior to when you intend to go to bed, don't watch screens, which tend to flood your eyes with stimulating blue light (TV, computer screens, or mobile phones).
- Set aside worries for the next day. If you are really plagued by worries, write them down and say to yourself, *"These things I will deal with tomorrow" (during the day!).*
- Try to establish a regular bedtime routine. For example, listening to a certain kind of relaxing music, taking a warm bath/shower, reading or listening to a non-stressful story, doing some gentle stretching or yoga, or doing some deep breathing and/or body

relaxation techniques. This is another associative technique that is helpful in promoting regular sleep.

- Once you are in bed, if you don't fall asleep within thirty minutes, don't stress about it. Simply get up and resume some of the relaxing activities above. Don't try to fight your sleep system. You won't win!
- Once you feel sleepy, try again.
- Physical issues like pain, indigestion, etc. can really interrupt sleep. Likewise, low mood and anxiety really reduce sleep quality and quantity. If this is what you are dealing with, it's important to discuss the issue(s) with your GP.

Now, if you have diligently tried all the above without success, talk to your GP. He or she may try you on a short course of medication to get you over the hump of sleeplessness. Beyond this, ask to be referred to a good sleep specialist, preferably one knowledgeable about concussions, in order to have a sleep study. Other issues unknown to you, such as sleep apnea, restless legs, sleep cycle shifts, Etcetera, may have been worsened or brought on by the concussion.

4.5 Sound and Light Sensitivities

Early on in the concussion, light and/or sound sensitivity may be dominant. Generally, these dissipate gradually as the individual recovers. Unfortunately, some individuals do continue to experience such sensitivities well after the concussion is thought to be over (i.e., the PPCS period).

<u>Light Sensitivity</u>
The human eye can respond to a huge range of light intensity, from hardly any light at all to painful levels of

illumination. Our eyes can make out at least some detail on an overcast night (approximately 0.001 lux) and see on a bright, sunny day (approximately 10,000 lux). We regulate this huge spread of light levels in a number of ways. As the light levels change in your environment, your peripheral autonomic nervous system regulates how much your pupils close down (aka constrict) or open up (aka dilate). But being able to cope with different light levels does not just happen at your eyes.

The brain is involved too. A part of the brain called the thalamus has a role in regulating how much visual information the brain takes in. Likewise, the superior colliculus helps control eye muscles and has a role in managing light. Finally, at the cellular level of the brain, interneurons modulate how much stimulation (including light) comes into an individual neuron. If there is dysfunction in any of these mechanisms, you will struggle to cope with the light stimulus.

When we are faced with an overly bright environment and all the above mechanisms are not up to the task, individuals necessarily fall back on wearing wide-brimmed hats or sunglasses, squinting or shielding their eyes, or, as a last resort, retreating into a dark room. Sunglasses can be particularly helpful in the early days of a concussion or for patients with severe light sensitivity. The colour of the glass is also important. In one study comparing grey tint to glasses with FL-41 tint (rose-like), individuals with severe light sensitivity (aka photophobia) much preferred the FL-41 tinted glasses.[5]

<u>Sound Sensitivity</u>
The technical term for sound sensitivity is hyperacusis. In the scientific literature, this term is used in many

different ways, including heightened sound awareness, sound hypersensitivity, sound hyperresponsiveness, sound intolerance, sound irritability, sound annoyance, sound pain, and phonophobia.[6] Landon and colleagues found that, in addition to attending to lower levels of sound and/or particular types of sound, TBI individuals with hyperacusis will also often consider these sounds annoying or threatening. Noise generated by others was more emotionally problematic than uncontrollable, more "natural" sounds. There is a negative feedback loop between hyperacusis and fatigue/concentration.[7]

Cognitive Behavioural Therapy (CBT) has proven effective for those suffering from prolonged or severe problems with hyperacusis.[8] Such treatments generally include: [9]
- education about the condition;
- relaxation and mindfulness techniques;
- moderating the degree of emotional reaction to the sound;
- challenging erroneous beliefs (e.g., hurt = harm); and
- graded exposures to different levels of sound, types of sound, sources of sound, and the environment.

The good news is that treatment is quite effective. The basic principles for reducing sensory sensitivity of both types are the same:
- As soon as possible, you are encouraged to reduce the use of devices that limit the intensity of the light or sound (e.g., sunglasses, earplugs, etc.) and not avoid noise unless it is very loud or you are very tired. It is important not to use these devices too much and to wean yourself from them. Otherwise, you will gradually increase your sensitivity.

- Gradually expose yourself to longer, then higher, levels of sound and/or light.
- Consult a professional if these sensitivities provoke strong negative emotions (e.g., fear) and/or impact the quality of your life (e.g., longer term avoidance behaviours). If this applies to you, talk to your family doctor and/or a qualified psychological counsellor. Graded relaxation and Cognitive Behavioural Therapy can be very helpful.

4.6 A DIY Approach to Relieving Sound and Light Sensitivities

<u>Sound Sensitivity</u>
In the early days of a concussion, sound sensitivity can be helped by a number of different strategies. Start with the following: turn down the volume, decrease the treble/heavy base of a sound system, avoid crowded/ echoey spaces, and use sound-reducing devices (e.g., earplugs).

<u>Sound-reducing devices</u>
- Earplugs. They come in off-the-shelf and custom-made varieties.
  - Moldable silicone earplugs (less sticky than wax earplugs) that cover the ear holes. Depending on the frequency you are hearing, these earplugs will reduce what you are hearing 22-37 dB.
  - Foam earplugs are inserted into the ear canal (not too far). Again, depending on the frequency you are hearing, these earplugs will reduce what you are hearing 36-50 dB.
  - Silicon earplugs with filters. These are more comfortable to wear and have the flexibility of allowing the user

to vary the amount of reduction. For example, Alpine Music Safe Pros have a white filter (16 dB), silver filter (19dB), and gold filter (22 dB).

Generally, foam earplugs are the best for reducing sound, particularly at higher frequencies. The custom-made plugs (foam and rubber) are more durable, fit the ear canal better, and have better performance. However, they are much more expensive.

- Earmuffs that cover the entire ear can better exclude unwanted sound, but they can be uncomfortable and hot to wear for longer periods.
- Noise-cancelling headphones have electronic ways of further reducing the sound. There's a variety of types. The most effective have active noise cancellation (ANC) technology, best used for situations where there is a constant and fairly loud background noise (e.g., travelling in a plane). Depending on the frequency, they can reduce sound up to 60 dB. However, noise-cancelling headphones have the same disadvantages as earmuffs and are also quite expensive.

Always choose the simplest option first. Avoid excluding too much sound, especially as this can be dangerous when walking in the community. Generally, for the first month, I recommend my patients use the simple foam earplugs. If, after a month, they're still struggling, they can purchase silicon insert earplugs with filters. This gives them a lot of safer choices. With these silicon plugs, please:

- Try not to use them at all (best option).
- Thereafter, use the filter that excludes the least amount of noise. Upgrade to a stronger filter only if necessary.

- Use the highest level of filter when you are very tired and/or in a very challenging environment.

<u>Exposure Exercises</u>
To help speed up sound desensitization, you can do one, or both, of these exercises:

- Graduated Sound Exposure. As you putter around the house, listen to music via headsets or earplugs. Systematically, over time you can:
  - Change the times of day you listen. Later in the day is harder and more tiring.
  - Start with just music, then add lyrics later. Language is harder for an overloaded brain to filter out.
  - Increase the length of time you expose yourself to the sounds.
  - Increase the volume of the music (do not approach maximum recommended decibel levels for a given time).
  - Increase the pitch of the music.
  - Increase how complex or discordant the music is (e.g., easy listening vs. hard rock).

- Sound Zooming. Like the eyes, your brain can pay attention (i.e., zoom in) to a particular sound and ignore other competing sounds (e.g., a particular person's voice in a crowded room). How this works is not well understood, but being able to triage sounds is an important skill, one initially quite difficult for concussed individuals. To speed the reacquisition of this skill, and to generally reduce sound sensitivity, try the following strategies.

Start in a relatively quiet place. As tolerated, focus in on sounds and conversations around you, close at hand and farther away. Just as with the sound exposure exercise, you should:

- o Change the times of day you go to these environments. Later in the day is harder and more tiring.
- o Increase your time in these environments.
- o Increase the volume and discordancy of the sounds to which you are exposed (e.g., a quiet bookstore with a few people versus a large food court at lunchtime).

This exercise has the added benefit of being a good mindfulness exercise to bring you into the here and now and to alleviate stress, depression, and anxiety.

<u>Light Sensitivity</u>

The process is very similar to sound sensitivity. The only significant difference is the devices used to initially lessen light exposure. These include:

- Sunglasses with anti-glare and UV protection. Try to use the minimum darkness of glasses you can manage. The less dark the glasses, the better. As you become less pained by light, use the sunglasses less and less and/or use lighter and lighter sunglasses, if you can find them.
- Experiment with the colour of the tint. There is evidence that the rose-like tint FL-41 can be quite helpful, especially for headaches and migraines.[5]
- Where possible, use: natural light rather than artificial light, task lighting versus overhead lighting, and incandescent/non-flickering LED over flickering fluorescents.

- Use screens that decrease the blue light output, or apply an external filter. Blue light will tend to stimulate your brain, making it hard to sleep, especially if you use the screen later in the day.
- Via apps (e.g., *f.lux* [10] and *Colorveil* [11]), change the balance or the dominant colour of the background from white to something more soothing.
- Purchase a low-flickering or a non-flickering monitor that employs e-ink technology (i.e., *Noviscend's* Iris Monitor [12]). The non-flickering monitor is generally as comfortable as reading paper. The downside is that it doesn't handle things like video well and is quite expensive. However, it can be very helpful when needed, especially if combined with a regular or low-flicker monitor for video.

4.7 Emotional Issues Are No Less Real

Over the years, many of the patients I have worked with (and unfortunately, some clinicians too) have believed that emotional issues associated with concussions are less real than their physical and cognitive difficulties. Thus, they blame themselves, or are blamed by others, for not being able to bring their emotions quickly under control. Somehow, they see it as a weakness of character.

Your brain is your headquarters. As such, you depend on it for everything from perceiving you have pain in your big right toe (and moreover, doing something about it) to managing your emotions. Trouble with emotions is sometimes discounted by the concussed person, and, very frequently, by those around them. People with a concussion or PPCS will often hear something like, *"For goodness' sake, just try to think more positively,"* or *"You're such a grump!"*

Even if you don't have a brain injury, controlling your emotions in this world can be a challenge. With a concussion, it is very hard indeed. Irritability, sadness, and anxiety are indeed as real and important—if not more important—for the concussed person as the more physical ailments such as neck pain, dizziness, and headaches. Generally, all a concussed person really needs is a bit more understanding, empathy, and, above all, patience, not only from those around them but, crucially, from themselves.

Sometimes, all the good will and effort in the world is not enough for a truly depressed and/or anxious person with a concussion or PPCS. They are, in a sense, at the bottom of a hole. Sometimes they are so deep in that hole that it doesn't matter how hard they try to jump—they are simply not going to clear the edge.

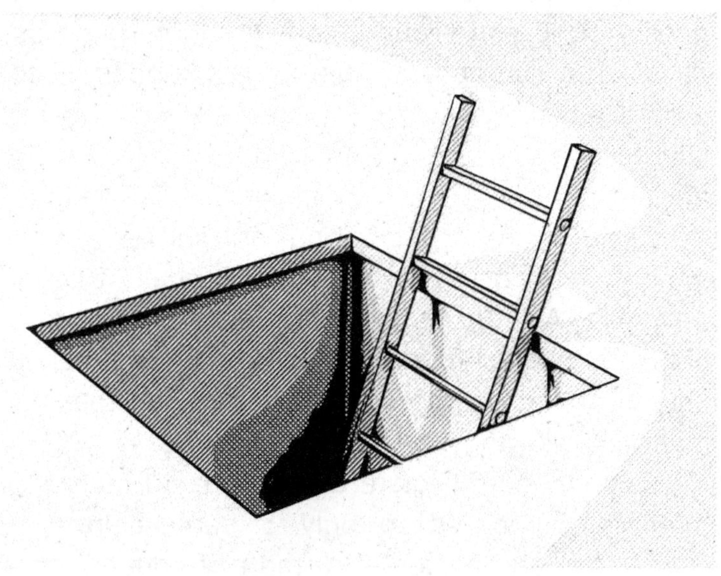

What they need is the help of a ladder. Thereafter, usually they can dispense with the ladder and go on their (at least somewhat) merrier way. The ladder they need is professional help, either in the form of counselling and/or from prescribed medication.

Counselling (aka talk therapy) and medications seem to work better together than either of them alone. So, if you or a loved one are in this situation, don't think of emotional problems as some great weakness on your, or their, part. There are many very good physiological and psychosocial reasons for the situation. More importantly, there is good help to be had. You should start by talking to your GP.

Like light and sound sensitivity, emotions and fatigue are entwined in a negative feedback loop. The more fatigued you are, the more you will struggle with your emotions. At the same time, the more you ruminate, the greater your difficulty in sleeping and resting effectively. Ruminating is like a race car that continues indefinitely. It goes around and around, consuming huge amounts of fuel. When it runs out of gas, it simply goes in, fills up, and off it goes again with its repetitive and unproductive thoughts.

Regardless of age, depression and anxiety are more common in concussed individuals than the general population. An analysis of a very large number of concussed children found they had a three times greater chance of being diagnosed with depression than average children.[13] Following a sports-related concussion (SRC), up to 20 percent of collegiate athletes have depression-like symptoms, compared to only 5 percent in a control group.[14] Anxiety issues are more frequently seen in concussions (mTBI) than in moderate and severe TBIs. It's hypothesised that the loss of consciousness and amnesia, associated with more severe TBI, somehow prevents the subsequent development of emotional deregulation.[15]

Pharmaceutical Treatments by Doctors

There are no medications formally approved for treating emotional difficulties associated with concussion. However, many MDs prescribe a number of off-label medications.[16] Consult your GP for more information about these (at times) helpful medications.

Non-Pharmaceutical Treatments

There is emerging evidence that a number of different drugless approaches can be quite helpful. These include:
- Cognitive Behavioural Therapy for insomnia (CBT-i) [17];
- Cognitive Behavioural Therapy (CBT) when brought on early in the recovery[18];
- Mindfulness-Based Stress Reduction (MBSR)[19]; and
- properly graded, low-risk activities (see chapter 3).[20]

A DIY approach to dealing with the emotional consequences of a concussion is beyond the scope of this book. Nevertheless, there are a number of things worth mentioning. It is not unusual to react to a concussion by being more emotional. Mood disturbances should not be immediately medicalized. It's normal to feel sad about lost opportunities and anxious about when one can return to normalcy. The concussed person's universe has just shrunk, and they want to know when they can leave this smaller room of existence.

Unfortunately, some concussion events lead to more prolonged problems, resulting in major long-term losses to the person's physical, mental, and emotional capacities. Mourning more significant losses is normal and healthy, but professional support is very helpful in these cases.

It is very important for the concussed person to have a sense of their emotional status and to not deny the emotional impact of the injury. Nor should they be hyper focused on it, as often the symptoms will take care of themselves. However, if the emotional disturbance seems to be lingering too long or getting worse, they may need to consult their family doctor and/or a psychological clinician.

The Hospital Anxiety and Depression Scale (HADS) is a valid screening tool for depression and anxiety in the community (i.e., not just for hospitals).[21] Dr. Phillip Snaith and Anthony Zigmond developed the HADS. It is a short, self-administered questionnaire to identify *possible* anxiety issues or depression (I prefer the term "low mood," as you need a clinician to diagnose depression). It is not a comprehensive evaluation, nor is suitable for all patients (e.g., psychiatric patients), but it's very helpful for flagging a possible issue(s).

A concussed patient can easily use the HADS to give themselves a sense of their "emotional temperature." For each question, you draw a circle around the number of the answer most closely resembling how you've been feeling in the past week. Don't take too long over your replies; your immediate response is best. Please note, the scoring is only valid if you have drawn a circle for each of the questions.

Tick the box beside the reply that is closest to how you have been feeling in the past week. Don't take too long over you replies: your immediate is best.

D	A		D	A	
		I feel tense or 'wound up':			I feel as if I am slowed down:
	3	Most of the time	3		Nearly all the time
	2	A lot of the time	2		Very often
	1	From time to time, occasionally	1		Sometimes
	0	Not at all	0		Not at all
		I still enjoy the things I used to enjoy:			I get a sort of frightened feeling like 'butterflies' in the stomach:
0		Definitely as much		0	Not at all
1		Not quite so much		1	Occasionally
2		Only a little		2	Quite Often
3		Hardly at all		3	Very Often

For a form you can copy, and score, see Appendix F or https://www.paulgodlewski.com/concussion-exercise-tools-and-appendices/.

4.8 When Not to Go It Alone

There are a number of reasons you may not want to go it alone. Maybe the prospect of doing these exercises by yourself is daunting, or you know, in your heart of hearts, that you're not likely to persist on your own. In both cases, I recommend, depending on the issue, that you consult the appropriate clinician experienced in dealing with concussions.

Reasons requiring the aid of healthcare professional(s) include:

- The sleep hygiene strategies are not helping you achieve a restful sleep. Consult your GP and ask if a sleep study is warranted.
- With the passage of time, there has been little in the way of change in your mood. If low mood lingers past approximately four weeks, don't wait longer to seek help.
- Even using the strategies above, your noise and/or sensitivity is not improving. Or the sensitivity is evoking strong emotions and avoidance behaviours. Consult an

audiologist familiar with concussions, plus or minus a psychological counsellor.

- If you have lingering or worsening anxiety or are low mood, consult a psychological counsellor and ask your GP if mood medication is warranted.

References

1. Shekleton J., et al. 2010. "Sleep Disturbance and Melatonin Levels Following Traumatic Brain Injury." Neurology 74, no. 21(May), 1732-1738. https://doi.org/10.1212/WNL.0b013e3181e0438b
2. Ouellet, M.C., Simon Beaulieu-Bonneau, S. and Morin, C.M. (2006). "Insomnia in Patients with Traumatic Brain Injury: Frequency, Characteristics, and Risk Factors." *J Head Trauma Rehabil. 21*(3)199-212. https://doi.org/10.1097/00001199-200605000-00001
3. Concussion Ontario. 2023. https://concussionsontario.org/. *Living Concussion Guidelines. Guideline for Concussion/Mild Traumatic Brain Injury and Prolonged Symptoms for Adults 18 years of age and older.* Ontario Ministry of Health. Ministry of Long-Term Care.
4. Carney, C. and Manber, R. 2013. *Goodnight Mind: Turn Off Your Noisy Thoughts and Get a Good Night's Sleep* Oakland. USA. New Harbinger Publications.
5. Digre, K.B. and Brennan, K.C. 2012 "Shedding Light on Photophobia." *J Neuroophthalmol.* 32, no. 1 (Mar): 68–81. https://doi.org/10.1097/WNO.0b013e3182474548
6. Tyler, R. et al. 2014. "A Review of Hyperacusis and Future Directions: Part I. Definitions and Manifestations," *Am J of Audiol.* 23, no. 4 (Dec), 402–419. https://doi.org/10.1044/2014_AJA-14-0010
7. Landon, J. et al. 2012. "Hearing Every Footstep: Noise Sensitivity in Individuals Following Traumatic Brain Injury," *Neuropsychological Rehabilitation,* 22, no. 3 (Jan)

391–407.
https://doi.org/10.1080/09602011.2011.652496

8. Jüris, L. et al. 2014. "Cognitive Behaviour Therapy for Hyperacusis: A Randomized Controlled Trial," *Behav Res Ther,* 54, (Mar), 30–37. https://doi.org/10.1016/j.brat.2014.01.001

9. Pienkowski, M. et al. (2014). "A Review of Hyperacusis and Future Directions: Part II. Measurement, Mechanisms, and Treatment," *Am J of Audiol.* 23 no. 4 (Dec) 420–436. https://doi.org/10.1044/2014_AJA-13-0037

10. f.lux. 2024. https://www.justgetflux.com/

11. East-tec. 2024. https://www.east-tec.com/colorveil/

12. Noviscend. 2024. https://noviscend.com/shop/iris-monitor/

13. Chrisman, S. P. and Richardson, L. P. 2014. "Prevalence of Diagnosed Depression in Adolescents with History of Concussion," *J Adolesc Health.* 54 no. 5 (May), 582–586. https://doi.org/10.1016/j.jadohealth.2013.10.006

14. Vargas, G. et al. 2015. "Predictors and Prevalence of Post-concussion Depression Symptoms in Collegiate Athletes," *Journal of Athletic Training.* 50, no. 3, 250–255. https://doi.org/10.4085/1062-6050-50.3.02

15. Marinkovic, I. et al. (2020). "Prognosis after Mild Traumatic Brain Injury: Influence of Psychiatric Disorders," *Brain Sci.* 10, no. 12 (Dec) 916. https://doi.org/10.3390/brainsci10120916

16. Rabinowitz, A. and Watanabe, T. 2020 "Pharmacotherapy for Treatment of Cognitive and Neuropsychiatric Symptoms after mTBI," *J Head Trauma Rehabil.* 35 no.1 (Jan-Feb), 76–83. https://doi.org/10.1097/HTR.0000000000000537

17. Lu, W., Krellman, J.W. and Dijkers, M.P. 2016. "Can Cognitive Behavioural Therapy for Insomnia also Treat Fatigue, Pain, and Mood Symptoms in Individuals with Traumatic Brain Injury? – A Multiple Case Report," *NeuroRehabilitation.* 38 no. 1, 59–69. https://doi.org/10.3233/NRE-151296

18. Ponsford. J, et al. 2016. "Efficacy of Motivational Interviewing and Cognitive Behavioural Therapy for Anxiety and Depression Symptoms Following Traumatic Brain Injury," *Psychological medicine.* 46 no. 5 (Apr),1079–1090. https://doi.org/10.1017/S0033291715002640

19. Azulay. J, et al. 2013. "A Pilot Study Examining the Effect of Mindfulness-Based Stress Reduction on Symptoms of Chronic Mild Traumatic Brain Injury/Postconcussive Syndrome," *J Head Trauma Rehabil.* 28 no. 4 (Jul-Aug), 323–331. https://doi.org/10.1097/HTR.0b013e318250ebda

20. Pedersen, B.K. and Saltin B. 2015. "Exercise as Medicine—Evidence for Prescribing Exercise as Therapy in 26 Different Chronic Diseases," *Scandinavian Journal of Medicine & Science in Sports.* 25, S3 (Nov), 1–72. https://doi.org/10.1111/sms.12581

21. Zigmond, A. S., and Snaith, R. P. 1983. "Hospital Anxiety and Depression Scale." *Acta Psychiatrica Scandinavica,* 67, no. 6 (Jun), 361-370. https://doi.org/10.1111/j.1600-0447.1983.tb09716.x

Chapter 5

Headaches, Plus or Minus Neck Issues

"Some pain you can distance yourself from, but a headache sits right where you live." Mark Lawrence

Cheat Sheet

5.1 How Amelia Overcame Headaches and Neck Pain

Amelia was involved in a motor vehicle accident, sustaining a concussion and whiplash. She recovered, due to her own efforts, along with the help from a chiropractor, PT, and some specialist intervention.

5.2 Red Flag Symptoms with Headaches

I've outlined red flag symptoms that might occur immediately after the injury or in the following days for which you need to immediately consult an emergency MD. There are other yellow flag symptoms for which you need to consult an MD as soon as possible.

5.3 There Are 150-plus Different Types of Headaches. No, Really—There Are

Headaches that come after a concussion are most

often labeled by the *International Classification of Headache Disorders* (ICHD-3) as either posttraumatic headaches (PTHA) or headache attributed to disorder of the neck.

5.4 Deep Dive: The Connection Between Headaches and Neck Injury

Here I provide a more detailed investigation of how neck injury often leads to headaches. Concussion and whiplash share a number of symptoms. As a result, whiplash symptoms may be blamed, in whole or in part, on the concussion.

5.5 Tests to See if a DIY Approach May Relieve Your Neck-Based Headache Issues

I provide you with some simple self-tests that will indicate whether exercises will likely help your neck-based headaches. In addition, these tests will help you assess whether you can do exercises on your own or should consult a physiotherapist.

5.6 A DIY Approach to Relieving Tension-Like and Neck-Related Headaches

Based on the results of the self-administered tests above, you will learn which exercises to do and how to do them.

5.7 When Not to Go It Alone

Apart from contraindications and cautions noted in Red Flag Symptoms with Headaches, there are a number of other reasons why you may not want to go it alone. Good practitioners have many tools at their disposal to help eliminate your headaches faster and more effectively.

5.1 How Amelia Overcame Headaches and Neck Pain

Amelia was stopped at a red light when her car was struck from behind by a cube van traveling at sixty km/hour. The delivery driver had been inattentive, focussing on his mobile phone map to find the location of his next pickup. At the time, Amelia was attending to her infant daughter Samantha in a rear child seat. The violent impact of the van on her car forced her body and head to rotate and move sideways. Her seat belt abruptly stopped the movement.

For a seemingly long period, Amelia felt extremely dazed. She then checked on her daughter who, much to her relief, appeared perfectly happy. Almost immediately thereafter, Amelia became aware of a moderate headache and neck pain. The headache seemed to originate in the left side of her neck and radiate up into the back of her head to her left temple and left eye. She noted that fogginess and dizziness came on later that day.

The police and emergency services attended the accident. At emergency, X-rays and a CT scan cleared her of serious injury. The ER doctor diagnosed her with a concussion and moderate whiplash. She was instructed to consult her GP as soon as possible. Her GP examined her and prescribed some painkillers. Her GP referred her to a local combined chiropractor and PT practice.

The chiropractor found she had severely limited mobility and pain in her neck, particularly in rotating to the left and extending her neck backwards. The chiropractor also noted tenderness and spasms in the muscles just below the back of Amelia's head (touching these muscles brought on a headache), along the muscles on both sides of her neck, her right shoulder, and down into her upper trunk on the right. Her headaches worsened with poor posture and anytime she had to run after her toddler.

Her PT found her dizziness was provoked either when her head rotated or if her head was held still and her body rotated from below on a rotary chair. This indicated that Amelia's dizziness, at least in part, was also coming from her neck. Finally, using a specialized laser headset, the PT found that Amelia had a very poor sense of where her head was when her eyes were closed.

Over the next six to eight weeks, her neck's range of motion, strength, and proprioception (i.e., your sense of self-movement, force, and position of different parts of your body) returned to normal. This was the result of the combined efforts of the chiropractor (doing manual therapy), the PT's dizziness treatments, and Amelia doing frequent home exercise (see below and chapter 6). An additional three weeks were needed to resolve most of the rest of her concussion symptoms, including her dizziness. The symptoms that took the longest to improve were her tension-like headaches. Despite no prior history of migraines, she unfortunately went on to develop them. She now gets migraines about twice a month and sees a headache specialist from time to time to adjust her medication.

5.2 Red Flag Symptoms with Headaches

It is especially important that you go to emergency (ER) after an injury, or anytime early on, if you experience any of the following "red flag" symptoms:

- Headaches along with fever, chills, nausea, weight loss, neck stiffness, nighttime pain and/or sweats
- Headaches with a sudden onset of visual changes, tingling of the face, and/or into the arms/hands
- Headaches with a sudden onset of bowel and/or bladder incontinence
- Headaches with weakness on one side of the face/body and/or sudden difficulty talking or walking
- Headaches that have a sudden change in their frequency or severity, especially those in patients over fifty years of age
- Headaches that increase suddenly and significantly with positional changes (e.g., going from standing to lying down)
- Headaches that come on with coughing, sneezing, and/or straining yourself (e.g., as part of a bowel movement or lifting a weight)
- Your headache gets significantly worse or is severe
- Headaches along with pain in one eye
- You develop arm or leg weakness
- You develop problems speaking
- You experience increased sleepiness with a headache
- Headache along with a sudden change in level of consciousness
- A strong headache that comes on within a couple of minutes (aka a thunderclap headache)
- Headaches with a substantial reduction in your neck's ability to rotate (i.e., less than forty-five degrees either to the right or left)

This is so that the emergency physician can rule out a number of things (e.g., a brain bleed) that may have resulted from the injury.

5.3 There Are 150-plus Different Types of Headaches. No, Really, There Are

This is according to *The International Classification of Headache Disorders* (3rd edition) (ICHD).[1] ICHD divides headaches into two main categories: primary and secondary. A primary headache is classified when the headache is considered the main or only problem. A secondary headache is one that results from some other condition. Headaches that come after a concussion or injury to the neck are therefore classified as a secondary headache. It's important to understand that a secondary headache is not any less of a problem to the individual than a primary headache. In broad strokes, individuals with concussion will often be diagnosed as having either having a post-traumatic headache (PTHA) or a headache attributed to a disorder of the neck.

Post-Traumatic Headache (PTHA) [1]
According to the ICDH, to have a PTHA, you need the following:
- It has to have resulted from a traumatic brain injury (which by definition includes all concussions), and/or from whiplash.
- The headache has to have come on within seven days of the accident or of regaining consciousness.
- It can include any primary headache that the person had before the concussion event (e.g., tension or migraine headache), but which has been significantly worsened by the injury and is again within the same seven-day window.

Most, but not all PTHAs can be thought of as either "migraine-like" headaches or "tension-like" headaches. For the purposes of this book, the distinction between a migraine-like PTHA versus a tension-like PTHA is too complex to get into. Although a person with a concussion or whiplash may predominantly have one or the other of these types, it's possible for them to experience both, as well as other headache types.

<u>Headache Attributed to Disorder of the Neck</u>
(aka cervicogenic headaches) [1]
The ICDH has a separate classification for headaches resulting from to injury to the head and/or neck (aka cervicogenic). Cervicogenic headaches are thought to come from injury to the soft and hard tissues in the neck referring pain, via shared nerves, to the scalp and skull. This type of headache usually, but not always, has the following features:
- The headaches must come on within seven days of a neck trauma.
- Pain most often starts in the neck and shoulders. From there, it travels to the back of the head and, at times, to the top of the head.
- The position or movement of the neck can worsen it.
- Nausea is rarely associated with this type of headache unless the pain is severe.

Looking at emergency patients diagnosed with a concussion (mTBI), Dr. J. van der Naalt and colleagues reported that headaches were the most common concussion symptom.[2] They further reported that 51 percent of patients with concussions developed post-traumatic headaches (PTHA) within two weeks of the injury. Following a review of the literature, Dr. T. Rebbeck (PT) and colleagues reported that, after neck pain, headaches were the second most common symptom (70-80 percent) in individuals with whiplash (aka whiplash associated disorder or WAD).[3] Bear in mind, not all neck pain is from whiplash. Whiplash has some characteristics unique to itself (see the Deep Dive following). Finally, Dr. H. Lew and colleagues reported that while most PTHAs fortunately resolve within six to twelve months of the injury, up to a third of patients can still suffer from PTHA for longer than one year after injury.[4] They also noted that women make up most individuals dealing with PTHA.[4]

There is obviously an overlap between PTHAs and cervicogenic headaches. Moreover, concussion and neck injury are often associated with each other. This results in headaches that can be coming from one or both conditions. I find treating both is the most effective course of action. I tell my patients that concussion and neck injury are like evil stepsisters. The two of them love to go to the ball and cause Cinderella (at the very least) a headache!

Headaches that follow a concussion or injury to the neck can present in many ways. The diagnosis of a headache is complex. If the headaches are moderate in severity, linger, and are negatively impacting your quality of life, you absolutely need to consult your GP. They will likely refer you to a specialist (i.e., a neurologist, physiatrist, etc.). There are other very effective techniques for relieving headaches beyond medication. For example, Mindfulness-Based Stress Reduction, meditation, etcetera (see chapter 4).

5.4 Deep Dive: The Connection Between Headaches and Neck Injury

To understand this better, let's briefly discuss the anatomy of the neck. A good way to think of the neck is as a set of seven blocks (your vertebrae) stacked one on top of the other. The smallest sits at the top, the largest block at the bottom. The head is like a large, heavy bowling ball placed atop this stack of blocks. This whole arrangement is normally held together tightly and securely by the neck's numerous joints, disks, and ligaments (tough fibrous material connecting one bone to another), and its muscles. There are thought to be three major sources of neck-based headaches (aka cervicogenic headaches). These are:

- Injury to the ligaments of the neck, especially the alar ligament
- Injury to the three upper cervical nerve roots
- Flare-up of preexisting conditions in the neck, like neck osteoarthritis (aka spondylosis)

The alar ligament, which attaches the skull bone to the top vertebral bone (aka C1), is very susceptible to damage in a whiplash injury. So too are the top three nerves (aka cervical nerve roots). The neck joints are very robust, but if they're already having problems like osteoarthritis, they are more prone to further damage during a whiplash incident. This is particularly the case with those structures at the top of the neck and near the base of the neck. If the neck muscles are weaker (more often in women than in men) and/or have less intrinsic flexibility (men more than women), then whiplash injury is much more likely. Whiplash (aka whiplash associated disorder—WAD) is believed to give an individual concussion-like symptoms in two ways:

- From pain related to injury of muscles, nerves, disks, ligaments, and joints. These pain signals travel along the nerves to give the person a headache at the back of their head and radiate upwards and forward.

- Misalignment of the joints and stretching of the ligaments changes the way the neck perceives its position in space (aka dysfunction of the proprioceptive system). This will contribute to the individual feeling dizziness (aka vestibular dysfunction, see chapter 6) and having problems moving their eyes accurately (aka visual dysfunction, see chapter 7).

Dr. C. Marshall and colleagues noted that concussions and whiplash share many of the same symptoms. Remember, not all neck pain is from whiplash. Modifying their table for clarity, I have prepared the following to indicate where concussion and whiplash overlap and differ: [5]

Shared by each condition*

CONCUSSION	WHIPLASH (WAD)
Headache	Headache
Neck pain	Reduced/painful neck movements
Nausea and Vomiting	Nausea and Vomiting
Dizziness	Dizziness
Balance problems	Unsteadiness
Blurred vision	Vision problems
Difficulty concentrating	Problems concentrating
Difficulty remembering	Memory problems

Unique to each condition

CONCUSSION	WHIPLASH (WAD)
Sensitivity to light	Shoulder pain
Sensitivity to noise	Reduced/painful jaw motions
Feeling slowed down	Numbness, tingling or pain in the arm or hand
Feeling "in a fog"	Numbness, tingling or pain in the leg or foot
"Don't feel right"	Difficulty swallowing
Fatigue or low energy	Ringing in the ears
Confusion	Lower back pain
Drowsiness	
Trouble falling asleep	
More emotional	
Irritable	
Sad	
Nervous or anxious	

(* Note: different names are used in the concussion and whiplash list for similar symptoms)

> I mostly agree with their "unique to each condition" list. However, in my experience, there are additional overlapping symptoms between concussions and WADs. These are:
> - Patients with WADs also have sleep issues and increased irritability.
> - Patients with concussions/PPCS also experience occasional ringing in their ears.
>
> Regardless, from this table, you can see how the source of symptoms can be so easily confused between concussions and whiplash. For this reason, I will always try to decide if whiplash is a contributing factor to a patient's concussion.

5.5 Tests to See if a DIY Approach May Relieve Your Neck-Based Headache Issues

If you have checked with your doctor and don't have any of the red flag symptoms (see above), you can proceed to the self-tests. These simple tests will suggest whether you need to do some exercises to help neck-based headaches. In addition, they will give you a sense of whether you can do these on your own or if you should be consulting a physiotherapist.

Test Group 1: Neck Active Range of Motion (AROM) Tests
Sitting up straight and without straining, test your neck's available range of motion in all the following directions. For each movement, make sure you are sitting up straight.

- Sitting with your back supported, rotate your neck to the right, then left, holding each for a few seconds. Avoid tilting your head to the side. A mirror is helpful to ensure you're moving properly.
- Next, side tilt your head bringing your ear towards your shoulder on the right, then to the left.
- Bend your head forward, trying to bring your chin to your chest.
- Finally, tip your head backwards to look at the ceiling.

For a video of this see
https://www.paulgodlewski.com/concussion-headaches/

For each direction, note if your range of motion is more limited than normal, and how much you can do (e.g., left rotation, approximately thirty degrees).

Which directions:

Note any direction where movement *worsens* your headache or neck discomfort. When noting your own symptoms for neck discomfort, use the following scale:

None = 0/5, Mild = 1/5, Mild to moderate = 2/5, Moderate to severe = 3/5, Severe = 4-5/5

Note the direction and degree of discomfort produced (e.g., left rotation 3/5).

Which directions:

Note any direction that makes you feel dizzy/off-balance, and how much (e.g., forward bend 2/5)

None = 0/5, Mild = 1/5, Mild to moderate = 2/5, Moderate to severe = 3/5, Severe = 4-5/5

Which directions:

You don't have to be super accurate with these numbers. But if you note them, after doing some exercises, you can check later to see if you have made any progress. This is a great motivator to keep doing the exercises.

Finally, note any direction that gives you numbness or tingling in your face, neck, arm, or leg.

Which directions:

Where you feel it (e.g., right forearm tingling):

If you're having these symptoms, you should get checked out by a qualified medical professional (e.g., an MD or PT). Noting these things down will greatly help them to help you.

<u>Test Group 2</u>: Neck strength and endurance tests

A. <u>Neck Flexion Endurance Test</u>
For this test, you will need a bed and someone to time you.

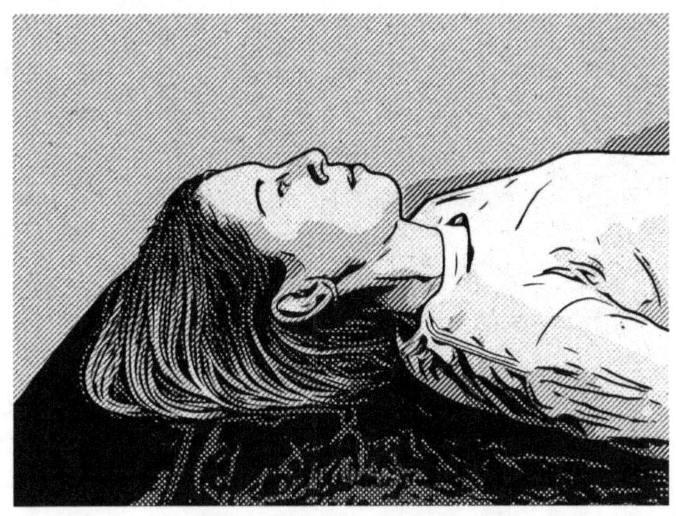

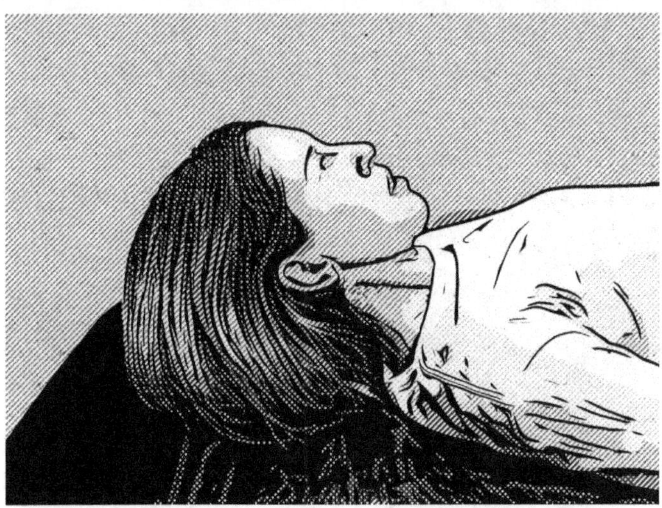

- Lie on your back, with your knees bent.
- Tuck your chin and keep your shoulders down, as you lift your head off the mattress or pillow.
- Stay in this position as long as you are able.
- Time how long you can do this and record this in seconds.

For a video of this see
https://www.paulgodlewski.com/concussion-headaches/

Stop the test if:
- you are unable to hold this position; or
- you can't keep your chin from poking up or your shoulders from raising up; or
- your head and neck start to shake a fair amount (a bit is fine); or
- your headache or neck pain is increased by more than a mild to moderate amount (i.e., 2/5).

There is a large variation in normal for this test. It depends upon your gender, age, and size. Normal for males is approximately 105-210 seconds. Normal for females is approximately 60-120 seconds.[6] It's best to consider yourself below normal only if you're significantly outside this variation and/or limited by symptoms.

B. <u>Neck Extension Endurance Test</u>
For this test, you will need a bed and someone to time you.

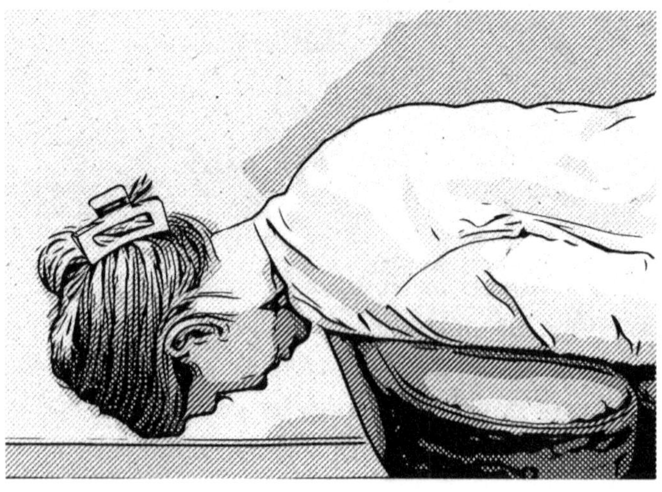

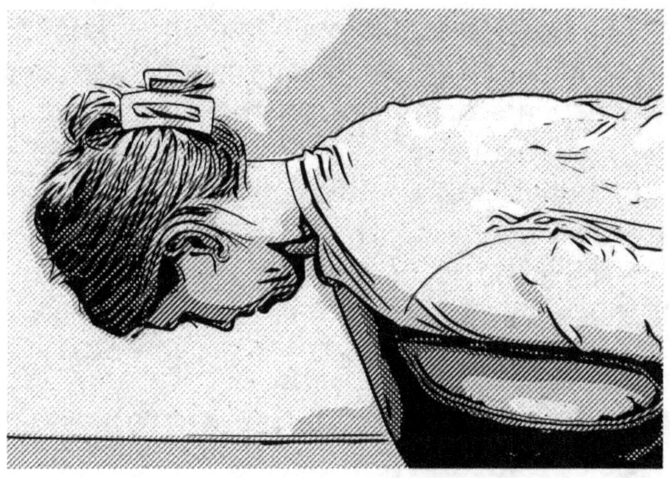

- Lie on your stomach with your arms straight back and your head & neck projecting beyond the bed.
- Keeping your shoulders down, tuck your chin, now lift your head to neutral and hold.
- Hold this position as long as you can. Time and record this in seconds.

For a video of this see
https://www.paulgodlewski.com/concussion-headaches/

Stop the test if:
- you are unable to hold this position without your head drooping/cogwheeling (i.e., your movements are jerky); or
- you can't keep your chin from poking downwards toward the table, or your shoulders from raising up; or
- your head and neck start to shake a fair amount (a bit is okay); or
- your headache or neck pain is increased by more than a mild to moderate amount (i.e., 0 to 2/5).

There is an even larger variation in normal range for this test, depending, again, upon your gender, age, and size. I advise patients doing this on their own to do just a simple neck extensor endurance test and to use a minimum criterion of 120 seconds to indicate weakness. In my experience, weakness in extensor muscles at the back of the head is fairly rare. If anything, in many people these muscles are often overly tight and strong.

5.6 A DIY Approach to Relieving Tension-Like and Neck-Related Headaches

If dizziness, neck pain, and/or headaches persist for more than ten days, the following exercises are recommended. With your test results in hand, you're ready to rebuild your neck's capacity. Fortunately for me, physiotherapy does not come in a pill form. Regularly exercising is an important factor in rebuilding your neck muscles' range of motion, stability, strength, and endurance. You need to do exercises twice a day for approximately six to eight weeks to see improvement. Initially, you only need to target those things you found problematic in your self-tests. But if you find these are not helping enough, or you wish to go further, you will need to consult a good local PT.

With all rehabilitation exercises, it's very important that you challenge yourself, as tolerated, by gradually increasing repetitions and difficulty level. Repeating the same exercise, without variation, will not build strength and endurance.

Try to work these challenges into everyday activities. If you don't practice these movements in real life, you'll have to get good at doing the exercises. Under the title "Day-to-Day Practices," I've included some examples. For all the exercises, make sure to keep a good, elongated, lying down/sitting/standing posture—as if you were a puppet and someone has pulled your centre string. Each time you do them, be sure to correct your posture. Sorry to say (sigh), but our mothers and grandmothers were right about the importance of good posture.

"Motion Is Lotion"

This is a very common saying, trotted out by physios since … since …well, as long as I've been a PT. It encapsulates an important concept: that, by its very nature, movement is necessary for healing in the body.

Neck Range of Motion (ROM) Exercises

The purpose of these exercises is to restore your neck's range, lubricate and provide nutrition to your neck joints, and normalize your neck's movements.

When to do this exercise:
These are all especially effective after a nice hot shower. But they're also effective at other times when your neck muscles are neutral in temperature. Do this exercise for any direction where the range of motion (ROM) is limited in test group 1 above. *Also,* where testing increases your symptoms (discomfort or dizziness) to no greater than two to three on a scale of five *and* does not bring on numbness or tingling in the face, neck, arm, or leg. If numbness or tingling does occur, don't do any of the following neck exercises before consulting an MD or good local PT.

This is the same movement as shown for the Neck active range of motion (AROM) tests above. Sitting in a chair with back support, move your head in the limited range. Hold for five seconds. Now add some gentle pressure with your hand pressing on your cheekbones. Hold for an additional five seconds. Repeat five times for each of the limited directions, two to three times a day.

Here is how to progress this exercise when you feel ready:
- Perform the exercise sitting without back support (e.g., sitting on a bed).
- Perform the exercise standing with your back supported (e.g., standing with your back, or side, against a wall).
- Perform the exercise standing without back support.

Day-to-Day ROM Practices
In your daily activities, try to make sure you're using as much of your range of motion as possible.

"Supple as a Cat"
Okay, so you've diligently done your range of motion, but each day you wake up and your neck is tight again. Why is that? Stretching for longer periods and repeating the stretches frequently, both when your muscles are warm (e.g., after a hot shower) and when cold, will more effectively help the muscles to elongate.
- Unless otherwise indicated, start doing the stretches by lying on your back, your knees bent. Taking gravity out of the picture will decrease the threat level and relax the neck muscles more.
- Unless otherwise indicated, do these exercises, if you can, without a pillow under your head.

- Do stretches two to three times a day, sometimes when the neck has been warmed by a hot shower or heating pad and sometimes when your neck is neutral in temperature.
- Hold all the stretches (unless otherwise indicated) gently at first for a *full* thirty seconds. (No cheating! Count "one thousand, two thousand … or one aardvark, two aardvarks . . ." Any multisyllabic animal name will do and help to pass the time. As an aside: I am sure aardvarks' mums love them, but I just happen to find them funny looking.)

Then, crank up the stretch a bit more for an additional *full* thirty seconds. Do not stretch to the point of discomfort. This is completely counterproductive to relaxing your muscles.

<u>Suboccpitals Stretch Exercise</u>
The muscles in the upper back of your neck, just below your head, are adjacent to many blood vessels and nerves. For this stretch, at least initially, you need to be a bit gentler and hold the stretches for shorter periods. Otherwise, you'll likely worsen your discomfort or give yourself a new headache.

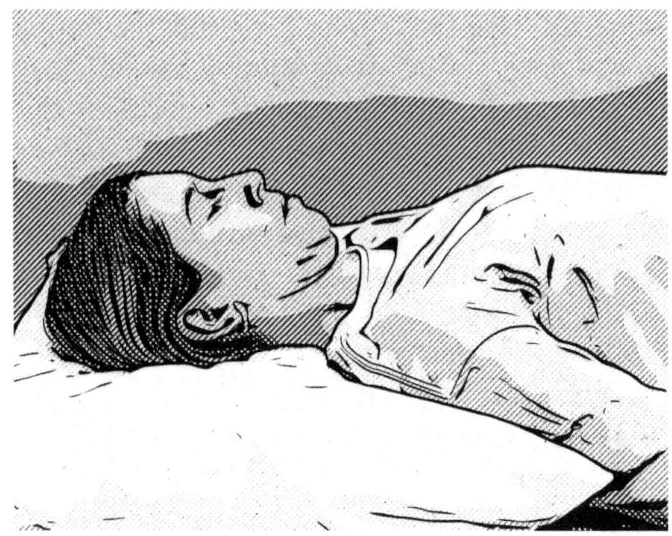

- Lie on your back with your head on a pillow and your knees bent.
- Push your head gently down into the pillow and tuck your chin a bit.
- Hold for five to ten seconds.
- Now, as tolerated, crank the chin tuck up a bit more.
- Hold this position for an additional five to ten seconds.

For a video of this see
https://www.paulgodlewski.com/concussion-headaches/

<u>SCM, Scalenes, and Upper Trapezius Stretch Exercises</u>
The muscles are located on the side of your neck. To stretch the left side of your neck muscles while lying on a mat or mattress, anchor your left arm under your hip. Hold this in three different positions:

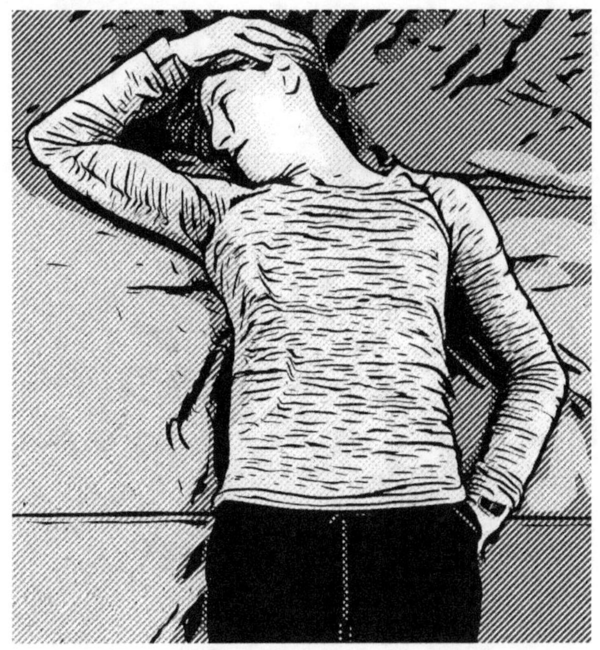

Head turned to the right and a bit downwards.

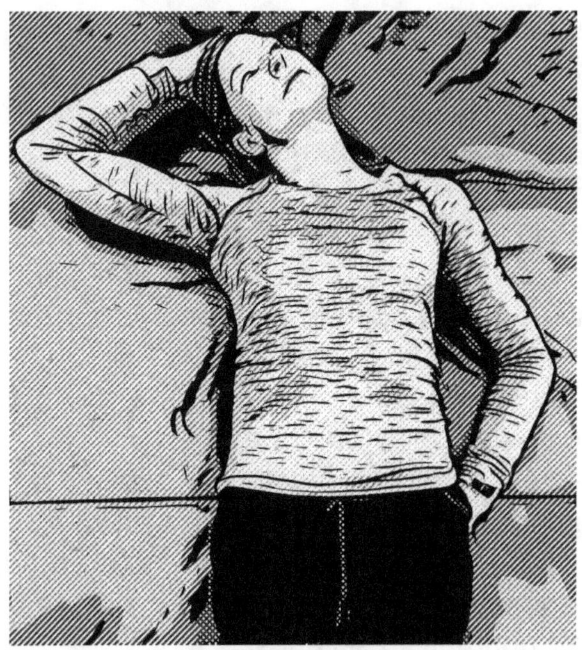

Head looking straight up to the ceiling.

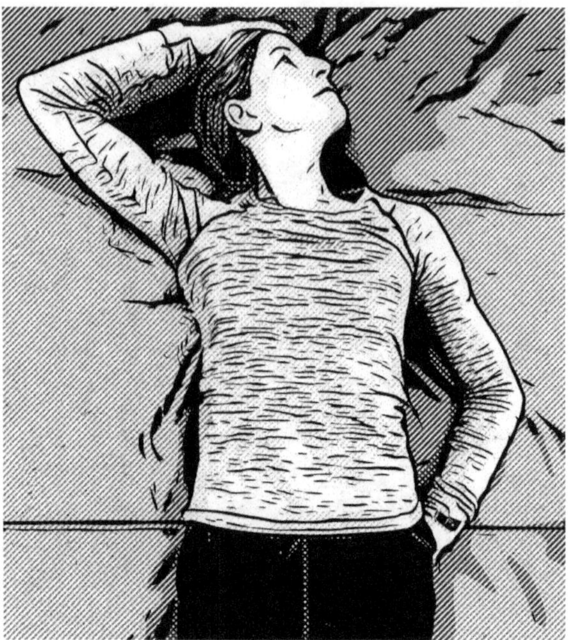

Head turned to the left and upwards.

- Lie on your back with your knees bent on a mattress or firm bed.
- For the left neck muscles, as shown, anchor your left arm and tilt your head right.
- To stretch all the muscle groups, you need to hold your head in three different positions:
- First, hold your head turned to the right and looking downwards. Now apply some gentle overpressure on with your right hand. Hold for 30 seconds. Then, as tolerated, apply some more pressure with your hand and again hold for 30 seconds.
- In this next variation, simply look straight up towards the ceiling. Apply gentle overpressure with your right hand. Hold for 30 seconds. Then, as tolerated, again apply some additional overpressure with your hand. Hold for another 30 seconds.

- In the final variation, tilt you head right, at the same time turning it to the left and looking upwards. Apply gentle overpressure with your right hand. Hold for 30 seconds. Then, as tolerated, apply more pressure and again hold for an additional 30 seconds.

Now do the mirror positions on the right side of your neck muscles.

For a video of this see
https://www.paulgodlewski.com/concussion-headaches/

<u>Paraspinal Extensors and Levator Scapulae Stretch Exercises</u>
The muscles are located at the back of neck and shoulder blade. Do this exercise while sitting. As shown, anchor your right arm under behind your back. Tilt your head to the left. Turn your head to the left and down. Apply gentle overpressure with your left hand.

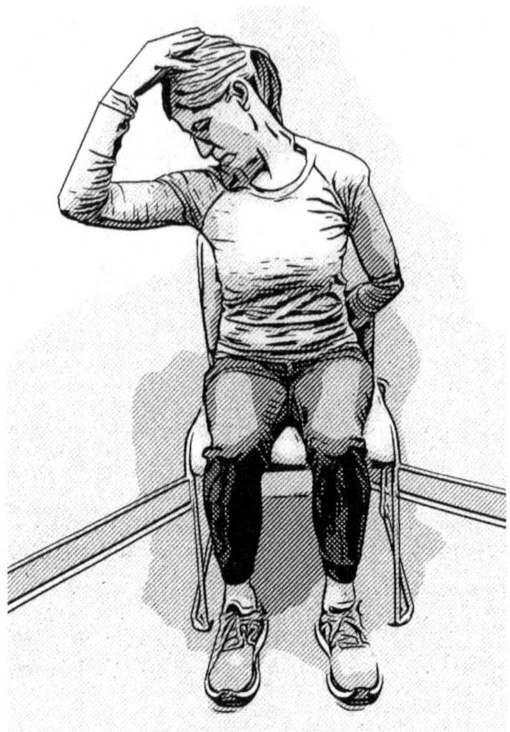

I irreverently call this "the-smelling-the-armpit" stretch.

- Do this exercise while sitting with your back supported.
- For the left neck muscles, anchor your left arm behind your back. Tilt and turn your head to the right and look downwards
- Apply gentle overpressure with your right hand. Hold for 30 seconds. Then a bit more for an additional 30 seconds.

Now do the mirror position on the right side of your neck muscles.

For a video of this see
https://www.paulgodlewski.com/concussion-headaches/

"Stable Like a Pyramid"

Joint stability is like having a good house foundation. Without a good foundation, the whole building would collapse in a storm.

Thus, in order for you to have strength in your fingers, you need adequate stability in your wrist. If your wrist is unstable, either because you had a bone break or inadequate joint and muscular stability, you simply won't have adequate strength in your fingers to grip or pick up objects. So too if you have inadequate stability in your elbow, your wrist can't do its job. This all works back, joint by joint, to your "core muscles," both in your neck and your trunk. Without adequate endurance, control, and stability of these deep neck core muscles, you simply don't have the ability to regain your neck's strength or range of motion and flexibility.

The body has a bit of a work-around, or "cheat" if you like, for this problem. If you lack adequate neck core stabilization, your brain will automatically substitute the big muscles of the neck and shoulder girdle to stabilize the neck. Unfortunately, Mother Nature has not endowed these large substitute muscles with the capacity to work for long periods of time. Without help from their small core muscle buddies, the big mover and groover muscles soon fatigue and develop their own exhaustion and pain. As if that's not bad enough, when large muscles are constantly "on," they end up unduly pulling on the neck and head's fascia (i.e., very thin ligamentous structures located throughout the body). This in turn will give you— you got it—more headaches!

Neck Stabilizing Exercises

The purpose of this exercise is to restore your neck's internal muscular stability. This is not the same as neck strength.

When to do this exercise:
I recommend you do this neck stabilization exercise for any neck injury. It helps to bring the deep core stabilizing muscles adjacent to your spine back online. Due to the injury, these have often gone quiet. At first, this exercise is a bit tricky as it requires you to feel the subtle contraction of your superficial neck muscles just under the skin.

Short Neck Flexors Stabilizers Exercise

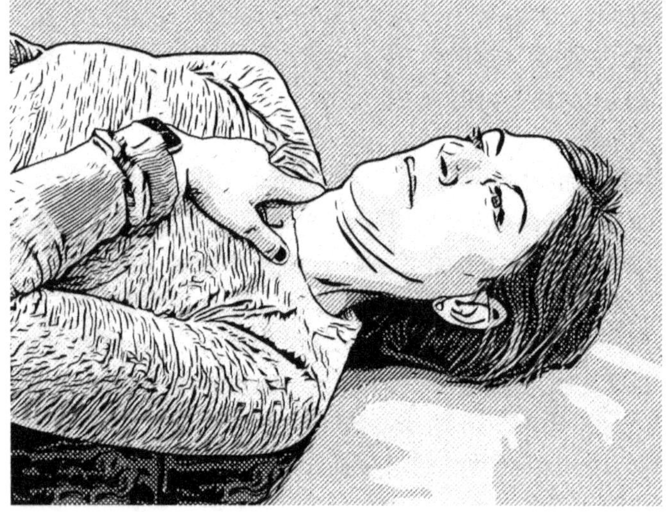

- Lying with your head on a pillow and knees bent
- Place your fingers on the muscles above your collarbone.
- Briefly lift your head off the pillow.
- You should feel the muscles strongly contracting under your fingers.
- Lower your head slowly back down.

The contraction you are now going to try to feel is the same, but much subtler. This time, without lifting your head off the pillow at all, tuck your neck very slowly and gently, as if you are giving yourself a small double chin.

- This time, without lifting your head off the pillow at all, tuck your chin very slowly and gently.
- With the tips of your fingers, try to feel when the muscles just begin to contract then back off.
- This should feel like a bowstring tensing

If you avoid turning on the superficial muscles but are still able to tuck your chin, it means the movement is coming from the short neck muscles that help to stabilize your neck. If the superficial muscles quickly come onboard, this means they are trying to make up for the lack of the stabilizers working well or enough. This in turn will lead to neck fatigue, soreness, and headaches. Your mission (should you choose to accept it) is to try to tuck your chin deeper and deeper without having the superficial muscles kick in.

For a very severe neck injury, a person may feel their superficial muscles kick in immediately. If this is the case, you just need to practice trying to look down toward your feet with your eyes alone, without getting the superficial muscles to contract. If, on the other hand, you are having no issues with this early outer muscle contraction, you will be able to give yourself a moderate double chin before you feel the superficial neck muscles kicking in. If so, don't worry about trying to feel the muscle contraction anymore. But to increase the strength and endurance of these neck stabilizers, just practice doing more repetitive neck tucks to this moderate double chin. Doing a deeper neck tuck is not a good idea.

Unfortunately, that is not the end of the story with respect to getting your neck back into shape following an injury. There are two additional parts. The first part involving the need to restore your neck's strength I will cover next. The second one, about the neck's proprioception (i.e., knowing where it is in space), I will briefly discuss in "Neck Gone Astray" (below). Mostly I will cover it (including—oh, goody!—more exercises) in the chapter about dizziness (see chapter 6). And you thought good physiotherapy was so easy-peasy!

For a video of this see
https://www.paulgodlewski.com/concussion-headaches/

"Strong Like a Bull"
"Hmm," you say, "as advised, I have now done my range of motion exercises, stretches, and stability exercises, and still my neck remains uptight and painful. So, what's up with that then, Mr. Physio?!"

Range, flexibility, and stability are important pieces of the puzzle, but strength of the muscular system is equally important. Look at it this way: there is little point in your neck becoming looser if it does not have the strength to hold and move your head (weighing in at approximately 4.5 kg or 10 lbs). The principle of "use it or lose it" applies throughout the body. If you haven't been using a certain part of your neck's range due to inflexibility and/or pain, you will very soon (in a matter of days!) start to lose strength in this range.

<u>Neck Strengthening and Endurance Exercises</u>
The purpose of these exercises is to restore your neck's strength and endurance. To some degree, they also inoculate you from getting a future whiplash and/or

concussion. In general, start with the gentle isometric neck exercises, especially if you are sore or your symptoms are quite reactive. Once these become easy and your symptom reactivity is reduced, go on to the more challenging neck strengthening and endurance exercises below.

<u>Isometric Neck Strengthening Exercises</u>
When to do these exercises:
If you find your neck strength is limited while performing any of the Test Group 2 (above), practise the following. While doing these exercises, the head and neck *don't* move. The neck muscles should only contract.

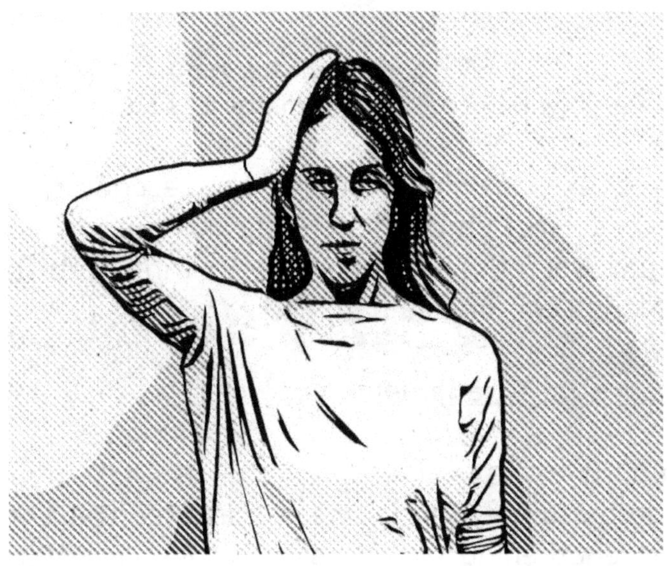

Challenge your neck to push without moving in the following directions:
- Start each movement with a good, elongated posture.
- Push your head into your resisting hand, gradually building up the pressure.

- Do not push so hard that it causes you head to move more than a little.
- Start with your hand on the right side of your head and resist your head rotating to the right.
- Repeat on the left.
- Again, place your hand on the right side. This time resist tilting your ear towards your right shoulder.
- Repeat on the left.
- Place both hands on your forehead and resist your head tipping forward towards your chest.
- Finally, place both hands on the back of your head and resist the neck tipping the head back to the ceiling.

For a video of this see
https://www.paulgodlewski.com/concussion-headaches/

For each exercise, hold for five full seconds (i.e., one aardvark to five aardvarks). Build doing each direction from one set of five repetitions to three sets of five repetitions, two times a day.

Neck Curl-Ups Strengthening Exercise

When to do this exercise:
Only go on to these if you have mastered the isometric neck strengthening exercises or if they were too easy from the start *and* didn't bring on too much discomfort and/or other symptoms. Do this exercise if your neck's strength is found to be below average in Test Group 2A above.

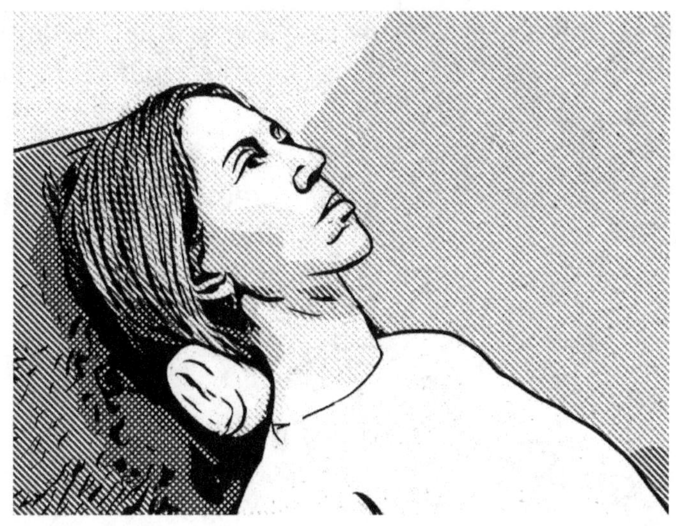

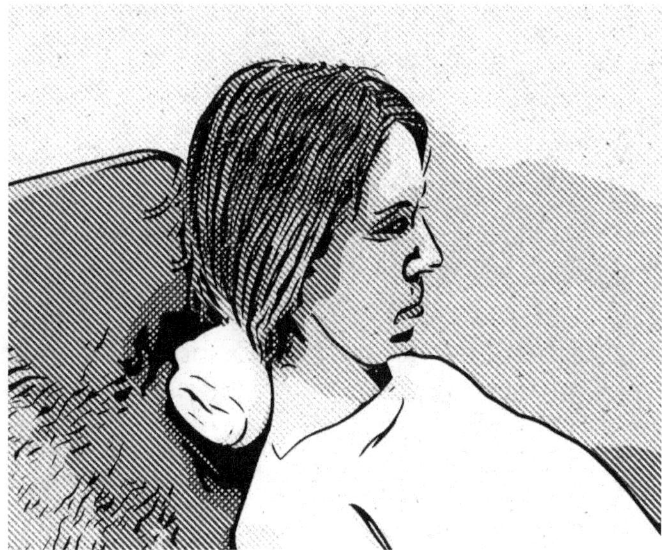

- Sit in a chair that can be inclined to different angles. Start at about seventy-five degrees. Place a towel roll in the small of your neck.
- Tuck your chin and keep tucked throughout. Slowly and smoothly curl your neck until your head is upright. Hold this for five seconds.

- Now slowly and smoothly lower your head back. Only when your head is fully supported should you relax the chin tuck.

Here is how to progress this exercise when you feel ready:

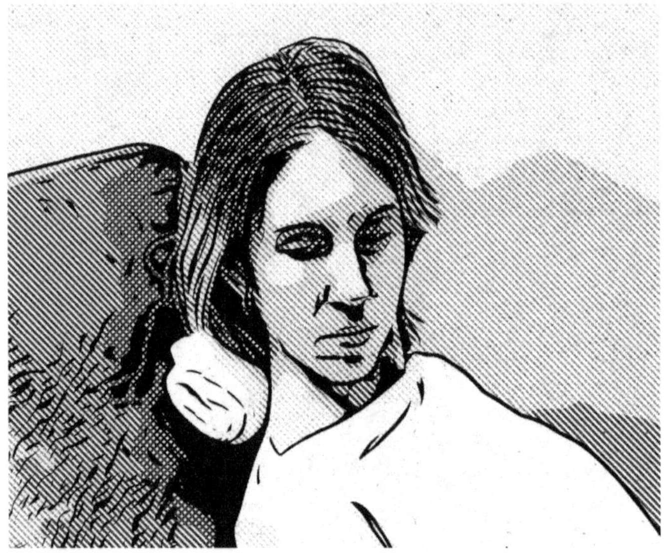

- With your head in the vertical position, turn your head to the right and left as far as you comfortably can.
- Maintain your chin tuck throughout and avoid tilting you head downwards.

Build from doing one set of five repetitions to three sets of five repetitions, two to three times a day. Over time, try to turn your head a bit further to the right and left.

For a video of this see
https://www.paulgodlewski.com/concussion-headaches/

Optimally, carry on lowering the incline angle until you can comfortably and easily do this exercise lying flat, raising your head as far as you can to the veritical and rotating left and right fully for three sets of five repetitions. Although you won't look the part, I tell my patients this exercise will make their neck as strong as an Olympic shot putter's.

<u>Neck Neutral Head Lift Strengthening Exercise</u>
Do this exercise if your neck's strength is found to be below average in Test Group 2B above. As shown, lie on a floor mat with a pillow under your chest, a towel roll under your brow, and your hands behind your back. Tuck your chin gently. Then raise your head to neutral and your arms upwards.

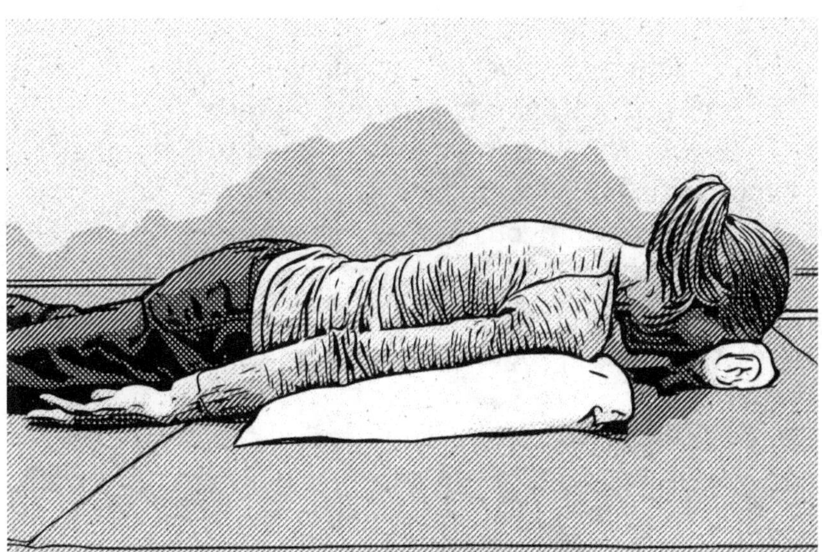

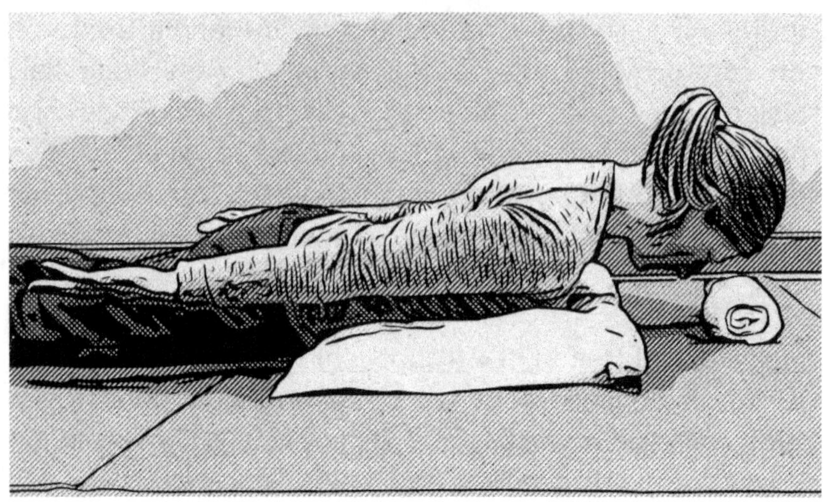

For a video of this see
https://www.paulgodlewski.com/concussion-headaches/

- With pillow and towel roll as shown, lie on a floor mat or firm bed with hands behind your back
- Tuck your chin. Then raise your head to neutral and your arms upwards.
- Do not overarch your lower back.
- Hold for 10 to 20 seconds. Lower slowly.

Here is how to progress this exercise when you feel ready:
Keeping your chin tucked and head in the lifted position (i.e., no drooping) throughout, turn your head to the left, then right, as far as is comfortable. Over time, gradually try to turn a bit further.

"An Ounce of Prevention ..."
It has been noted that women make up a disproportionately large percentage of concussion patients and go on to have longer-term symptoms (i.e., PPCS). One theory is

that this is because they have less robust necks than men. Thus, in the event of an accident, they get exposed to more acceleration-deceleration damage to both the neck and the brain itself.

Somewhat tongue in cheek, I suspect this is evidence of evolution in action. Men have been hitting each other over the head (and elsewhere) for so long now that perhaps only those with more robust necks and concussion-resistant brains have gone on to sire children. Joking aside, having a stronger neck, in general, is thought to be preventative of future concussion and whiplash injury, particularly for girls and women.

"Neck Gone Astray"

How precisely does a neck go astray—or, in other words, get lost? Isn't it permanently attached to your body and head? The answer is by the neck not knowing where it is. The body's capacity to know without looking where its various parts are is called proprioception. For example, because of proprioception, you can easily touch the tip of your nose regardless of whether your eyes are open or closed. Without it, eyes closed, you could poke yourself in the eye. The neck structures are very richly gifted with proprioceptive sensors. This is good because, in general, neck joints have a very poor tolerance for moving out of their safety zone. After all, they are protecting both the brain and the spinal cord.

In chapter 6, I will discuss how this contributes to dizziness in concussions and how, with simple tools, you can find out if you have poor neck proprioception, and how to rehab it. Even if you are not experiencing dizziness, this is well worth a read as an aid to getting rid of your headaches.

Other "Simple Tools"

To bring down swelling and pain in a knee, I use a simple device called a "Cryocuff." This device surrounds a swollen knee joint in a sleeve of very cold, pressurized water. Such simple tools, used at the right time, can also greatly relieve headaches or stop them from worsening.

For example, the judicious application of ice and heat can be very helpful. When it comes to necks, as with most of the rest of the body, the general rule of thumb I use is that cold is best applied in the first seventy-two hours of an injury. It reduces damage, suppresses inflammation, and acts as a local anesthetic for the nerves.

However, you need to be a bit careful not to overchill tissue. For this reason, the smaller the body part, the shorter the time you apply the cold. The goal is to get the target tissue area a bit numb. Once the tissue has reheated itself, say in an hour or two, you can reapply the cold. For very small areas, consider giving the area an ice massage by rubbing it with an ice cube partially wrapped in a paper towel (the latter for the sake of your poor fingers).

After seventy-two hours, the general rule of thumb is that heat is best (but if you find cold more helpful, stick with that). It allows tight structures (e.g., muscles) to be stretched out and improves circulation, thereby improving healing. Unlike ice, so long as you use common sense (e.g., not having it too hot or sleeping on the heat source, etcetera), you can apply heat for long periods. Check your skin from time to time to see how it's doing.

Important Note: Do not use heat or ice in a given area if you have sensory loss there.

These recommendations are believed to hold true for both tension-like PTHA, where muscle relaxation is helpful, as well as migraine-like PTHAs. In 2013, Dr. A. Sprouse-Blum and colleagues found that participants applying a cold neck wrap at the onset of their migraine experienced significantly less pain thereafter. They hypothesized that this was due to the chilling of the blood in the carotid arteries at the front of the neck.[7]

I generally recommend that heat and ice be applied to the neck rather than the head. But many of my patients swear by the quick application of these, particularly ice, where their head hurts at the onset of their headaches. This is likely because the scalp, like the neck, is very rich in blood circulation, nerve endings, fascial structures, and muscles that benefit from its application. Just remember not to keep it on too long (see above) as the scalp's tissues are thin.

5.7 When Not to Go It Alone

Apart from cautions and contraindications noted in "Red Flag Symptoms with Headaches" (Section 5.2) above, there are several other reasons why you may not want to go it alone. If the prospect of testing or doing these exercises by yourself is daunting or if you know in your heart of hearts that you are not likely to persist on your own, I recommend you consult a good local clinician (e.g., a physiotherapist).

What is a good physiotherapy? While soothing modalities are at times helpful, just slapping on some electrical modality's electrodes plus an icepack or heat pack is not good physiotherapy! If this is all you are getting, (plus a few exercises if you are lucky), I suggest you look elsewhere for better quality therapy.

References

1. Olesen, J. et al. 2018. "The International Classification of Headache Disorders, 3rd edition." *Cephalalgia,* 38, no. 1, 1–211. https://doi.org/10.1177/0333102417738202
2. van der Naalt, J. et al. 2017. "Early Predictors of Outcome after Mild Traumatic Brain Injury (UPFRONT): An Observational Cohort Study." *The Lancet Neurology* 16, no.7, 532-540. https://doi.org/10.1016/S1474-4422(17)30117-5
3. Rebbeck, T. et al. 2019. "Concussion in Combination with Whiplash-Associated Disorder May Be Missed in Primary Care: Key Recommendations for Assessment and Management." *Journal of Orthopaedic & Sports Physical Therapy* 49, no. 11 (Oct) 766-867. https://doi.org/10.2519/jospt.2019.8946
4. Lew, H. L. et al. 2006. "Characteristics and Treatment of Headache after Traumatic Brain Injury: A Focused Review." *American Journal of Physical Medical and Rehabilitation 85*, no 7 (Jul), 619-27. https://doi.org/10.1097/01.phm.0000223235.09931.c0
5. Marshall, C.M. et al. 2015 "The Role of the Cervical Spine in Post-Concussion Syndrome." *Phys Sportsmed* 43 no. 3 (Jul), 274–284. https://doi.org/10.1080/00913847.2015.1064301
6. Kennedy, C. 2015. PT Postgraduate course "Concussion, What About the Neck?"
7. Sprouse-Blum, A. S. et al. 2013 "Randomized Controlled Trial: Targeted Neck Cooling in the Treatment of the Migraine Patient." *Hawaii J Med Public Health* 72, no. 7 (Jul), 237–241. https://pubmed.ncbi.nlm.nih.gov/23901394/

Chapter 6

Dizziness, Vertigo, and Imbalance, Plus or Minus Neck Issues

"It's like standing on the deck of a ship in really high seas." Laura Hillenbrand

---

Cheat Sheet

6.1 How Nia Overcame Dizziness and Neck Pain

Nia's concussion and whiplash resulted in immediate and significant dizziness, disequilibrium, and brain fog. It required a lot of patience and perseverance to do her exercises and recover fully.

6.2 Red Flag Symptoms with Dizziness

I outline a number of red flags that indicate you should go to the ER at your local hospital. This is so that the emergency physician can rule out a number of serious issues (e.g., a brain bleed).

6.3 Potential Sources of Your Dizziness

I broadly outline the large number of sources for dizziness. Although concussion is the most likely reason for your dizziness, don't assume that your dizziness is only concussion-related.

6.4 What Are Dizziness and Vertigo?

When it comes to dizziness, people use a large number of descriptions. In medicine, vertigo is a special kind of dizziness, one that requires you to experience the illusion of movement.

6.5 Concussion-Related Sources of Dizziness

There are a number of sources that are concussion-related dizziness, which I list. I go into more detail about one source of vertigo and dizziness: benign paroxysmal positional vertigo (BPPV).

6.6 Deep Dive: The Connection Between Concussion and Dizziness

I explain how your balance systems normally work to prevent dizziness, keep your head and body upright, and maintain your balance. I briefly describe how this normal functioning can be disrupted by a concussion and other associated issues (e.g., whiplash).

6.7 Tests to See if a DIY Approach Is Likely to Relieve Dizziness and Imbalance

These tests will tell you which exercises you need to do. They will also give you a sense of whether you can do this alone or need help from a clinician.

6.8 A DIY Approach to Relieving Dizziness and Imbalance

With your test results in hand, you are ready to work on your dizziness and disequilibrium. Be gentle, patient, and persistent. It will take you some time to reduce your symptoms.

> **6.9 When Not to Go It Alone**
> Apart from red flags noted in Section 6.2 above, I outline a number of other reasons why you may not want to go it alone.

6.1 How Nia Overcame Dizziness and Neck Pain

A manager with a large company, Nia was returning home from a business trip. The long trip home had been made even more trying by severe weather delays. By the time her plane had been given permission to land, all the passenger boarding bridges were mired in snow. Passengers needed to disembark via a stair to a bus waiting to take them to the terminal. Unfortunately, the bus jolted very hard while going over a ridge of snow. A heavy suitcase came free from an overhead cage and struck Nia on the right side of the head. She lost consciousness, but just for a few minutes.

On waking, she experienced immediate and significant dizziness, neck pain, and problems with her balance, so much so that she needed assistance to walk. Nothing abnormal was found with any of the tests done at the local hospital. The ER doctor diagnosed Nia with a concussion and discharged her to the care of her family doctor. On examination later, her GP additionally diagnosed her with whiplash and referred her to an otolaryngologist (aka an ENT specialist). Her GP also referred Nia to a local chiropractor. The chiropractor suspected that, while some of the dizziness seemed to be coming from the neck (aka cervicogenic dizziness), much of the dizziness appeared to be concussion related.

He therefore referred Nia to a vestibular physiotherapist colleague, who was also experienced in concussion management. In time, the specialist ENT diagnosed Nia with a labyrinthine concussion.

These two clinicians worked together, the chiropractor dealing with her neck issues and the PT the vestibular and concussion issues. One day, while getting up from one of the chiropractor's treatments, Nia experienced a very strong but brief (approximately thirty seconds) bout of visual spinning sensation. Realizing this was very likely benign paroxysmal positional vertigo (BPPV), the chiropractor instructed her to consult the vestibular physiotherapist.

Her vestibular PT found Nia had indeed developed a secondary case of right ear BPPV. The PT treated her with the appropriate maneuver, clearing her of it in just two sessions. Under the chiropractor's care, her neck symptoms and headaches resolved in three months. Unfortunately, her concussion-related symptoms of ongoing dizziness and brain fog took much longer to resolve. She persevered with her home exercises, and her patience eventually paid off. All told, it took Nia eighteen months to return fully to her demanding managerial work and travels.

6.2 Red Flag Symptoms with Dizziness

You need to consult your family doctor. In addition, it is especially important that you go to the ER if, soon after an injury, you experience any of the following "red flag" symptoms with your dizziness:
- You have nausea and/or vomiting.
- You develop facial, arm, or leg weakness.

- You develop double vision.
- You develop problems speaking.
- You develop sudden hearing loss.

This is so that the emergency physician can rule out a number of issues (e.g., a brain bleed) that may have come from the injury.

6.3 Potential Sources of Your Dizziness

Dizziness comes from a large number of conditions. Some of the many things that give rise to dizziness include:
- Medication
- Vestibular system disorders of the inner ear
- Neurological dysfunction
- Post-traumatic dizziness, including concussions (aka mild traumatic brain injury - mTBI).
- Neck issues
- Visual deficits
- Cardiovascular issues
- Psychological problems (at times, anxiety and depression can lead to dizziness)

Don't assume that the dizziness you feel after the injury is just coming from your concussion. This may or may not be the case. Initially, always consult your GP.

6.4 What Are Dizziness and Vertigo?

How you perceive dizziness seems to depend more on you than the condition that is bringing it on. The kinds of description patients use include feeling faint, woozy, lightheaded, a feeling of heaviness at the back of the head, weak in the knees, unsteady, tilting, rocking, floating, walking on spongy floors, etcetera. Alone or in combination, all of these are used by people to describe the very big family of dizziness. While certain descriptions tend to come from certain conditions (e.g., light-headedness, where the heart is concerned), the type of sensation you have is not a reliable way to determine its origin.

A special note about vertigo. Vertigo is a term we use loosely in our day-to-day language that essentially means "dizzy." In medicine, however, vertigo properly used has a very specific meaning. To have vertigo—along with dizziness—you must experience an illusion of movement. Vertigo is an illusion of movement, either of the external world revolving around the person or the individual revolving relative to the space.

Depending on the source of vertigo, it can last for seconds or hours. It is often caused by positional changes of the body, but not always. Although some clinicians may use it this way, "vertigo" is *not* a diagnosis (one of my pet peeves!). It is just a symptom, as it can come from a variety of sources. What is causing the vertigo forms the diagnosis.

6.5 Concussion-Related Sources of Dizziness

There are many possible sources of dizziness, but most are fortunately rare. Generally, to tease these apart, you need a medical specialist called an otolaryngologist (aka an ear, nose, throat specialist or ENT) and/or a vestibular physiotherapist. With one exception, I'm not going to discuss these in any detail because of their complexity.

They include: [1,2]
- Post-traumatic dizziness (e.g., from a concussion)
- Labyrinthine concussion (aka vestibular concussion)
- Post-traumatic vestibular migraines (PTVM)
- Benign paroxysmal positional vertigo (BPPV)

For our purposes later in the book, this is worth expanding on a bit. Let's first break down the BPPV name:
- Benign - it is not going to harm you. (Oh good! Still, it can be a pain in the neck.)
- Paroxysmal - it comes and goes. Sometimes, in fact, it can fully fix itself without any help.
- Positional - it results from positional changes of the body or head (e.g., turning in bed, getting up or getting into bed, looking up at a shelf or downwards at a shoe). This form of vertigo doesn't happen when you just turn your head quickly, though you may feel briefly dizzy and off-balance.
- Vertigo - the illusion of movement (see above) of the environment around you or you in the environment.

Depending on the age of the person, BPPV is the most common source of vertigo and dizziness for the general population (approximately 30 precent). It is therefore the "go-to-diagnosis" (sometimes erroneously) for many clinicians. Traumatic BPPV is less common (15 percent) than nontraumatic BPPV. This is regardless of the kind of traumatic brain injury involved. [3]

Looking at how individuals who are concussed and have dizziness have done over time, studies have found:
- Those with vestibular ocular reflex (VOR) problems (see the Deep Dive below) will take longer to recover

and will have a higher risk of reinjury than those without. [4]
- Those who still have dizziness six months after their injury are more likely to recover less well overall and more slowly. [5]

<u>Specific to Sport-Related Concussion</u> (SRC)
- You are more likely to experience vestibular symptoms if you are female and/or had on-the-field dizziness, experience fogginess, or have post-traumatic migraines. [6]
- A large number of concussed athletes (50–84 percent) report dizziness. But when the vestibular system is specifically examined with a high-tech test, only 3 percent to 21 percent have any problems.[7] This means that the dizziness they are experiencing is most often *not* from damage to the inner ear's nerves. However, this study does not rule out other forms of damage to the inner ear. In approximately 60 percent of athletes, there are problems with the vestibular ocular reflex (VOR) and oculomotor problems. [7]
- A study by K.J. Schneider and colleagues showed that concussed individuals with dizziness, neck pain, and/or headaches were able to return to sports sooner if they were treated with a combination of neck physiotherapy and vestibular rehabilitation therapy (see below).[8]

6.6 Deep Dive: The Connection Between Concussion and Dizziness.

In order to make your way around your environment, your brain takes in information from a number of your senses. One of the other things your vestibular system does in your inner ear is maintain the stability of vision (aka the vestibular ocular reflex or VOR). Without a vestibular system, your vision would be more like an amateur film—jittery and out of focus— than one shot by a professional.

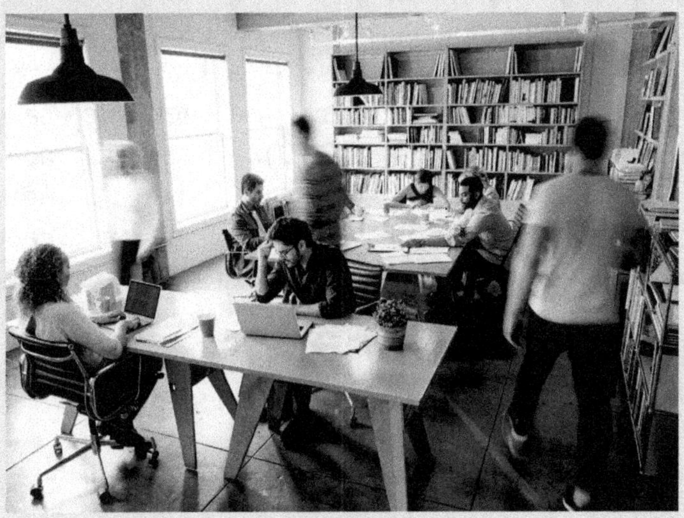

How do you think that would make you feel? Yup, in very short order, you'd feel dizzy and off-balance. If strong or lasting long enough, it would make you feel nauseous and cause you to vomit. For this reason, people with a badly working vestibular system or a concussion are usually also, quite sensitive to movement, especially within busy environments (e.g., grocery stores and shopping malls).

Dizziness and imbalance can also occur when there is a mismatch between one or more of your senses, giving your brain contradictory information. However, they can arise even if there is no problem with the information coming from these senses. As we saw in chapter 1, concussions can lead to issues at the cellular level. These problems can introduce errors and delays in the timing of the brain's thinking. The result is the same: dizziness, an "off" feeling, imbalance, motion sensitivity, and nausea.

How problems specifically at the neck level (e.g., whiplash) lead to dizziness is a bit complicated. Dizziness originating from the neck is called cervicogenic dizziness (CGD). "Cervico" means "relating to the neck," and "-genic" means "generated from." The capacity we all have called "proprioception" tells us where our body's parts are and how we are moving them. For example, you can touch your nose with a finger with or without your eyes being open because of proprioception.

Your neck is full of joints (twenty-eight to be precise!) similar to your finger joints. In cervicogenic dizziness (CGD), problems from injury (e.g., whiplash) or disease in the joints (neck arthritis) are thought to result in incorrect information being delivered to the brain. This leads to a mismatch between what your vestibular system is saying and what the neck is saying. This, in turn, leads to dizziness, poor balance, and reduced eye control (aka gaze instability).

Someone with CGD will report many of the following symptoms: [9]
- Dizziness
- Neck pain
- Neck stiffness or limitations in how far they can move their head
- Unsteadiness (standing and/or moving)
- Blurred vision
- Mild difficulty swallowing, ringing and other sounds in the ears
- Headaches (in my experience, most often in the back of the head)

Symptoms can be brought on with more neck movement, increased fatigue, stress or anxiety, and, in my experience, poor sitting or standing posture (e.g., working at the computer).

Individuals with CGD will generally **not** report:
- Severe headaches, double vision, facial numbness, difficulty speaking, or significant difficulty with swallowing. If any of these symptoms are present, go to emergency ASAP!
- Auras (sensory hallucinations)
- Fullness in their ears (i.e., the feeling you get going up a mountain)
- Hearing loss
- Medically defined vertigo (the illusion of movement, like visual spinning outside of you)
- Noise and light sensitivity

An experienced clinician will likely find a number of the following signs:[10]

- Tenderness in the neck muscles, particularly those just below the head (aka suboccipital muscles)
- Poor static and dynamic balance
- Reduced neck range of motion, both active and passive
- Poor neck stability, strength, and proprioception
- Gaze instability, but not nystagmus (i.e., involuntary rhythmic motion of the eyes)

CGD is not nearly as common as other forms of dizziness. For this reason, the condition is often diagnosed by making sure it isn't something else. While I understand the thinking behind this, different sources are not at all easy to tease apart. Therefore, I will always look for and often treat possible CGD-like issues, especially in the case of concussion and its evil stepsister, whiplash (see chapter 5, section 5.5, "Deep Dive: The Connection Between Headaches and Neck Injury). As with headaches, many of these symptoms are also seen in concussions by themselves. Therefore, don't assume that because you're ticking a number of these symptoms off in your mind, your dizziness and other symptoms are all neck related. Instead, consult a professional!

6.7 Tests to See if a DIY Approach Is Likely to Relieve Dizziness and Imbalance

If you have been checked by your doctor (see section 6.3) and/or by a physiotherapist to ensure you don't have anything serious wrong with your neck, you can proceed to the next steps to test yourself. The following simple test will indicate which of the exercises in the next section you will need to do to reduce your dizziness. In addition, it will give you a sense of whether you can do these on your own or if you should really be consulting a vestibular physiotherapist.

Test 1: Benign Paroxysmal Positional Vertigo (right side shown) Remember: not all dizziness is vertigo, nor does all vertigo come from Benign Paroxysmal Positional Vertigo (BPPV). Vertigo, especially from BPPV, must involve an illusion of movement happening outside of you (e.g., the room spinning). If the vertigo is coming from BPPV and not some other source, it will last no more than about two minutes, very often much shorter. However, you may feel dizzy on and off for a prolonged period after this. But just feeling dizzy while doing these tests *does not mean* you have vertigo!

Start by sitting on your bed with your legs stretched out in front of you. Place one to two pillows behind you (use one pillow if you have limited ability to bend your neck backwards). To test the right side, perform the following modified Dix-Hallpike maneuver (m. DH).

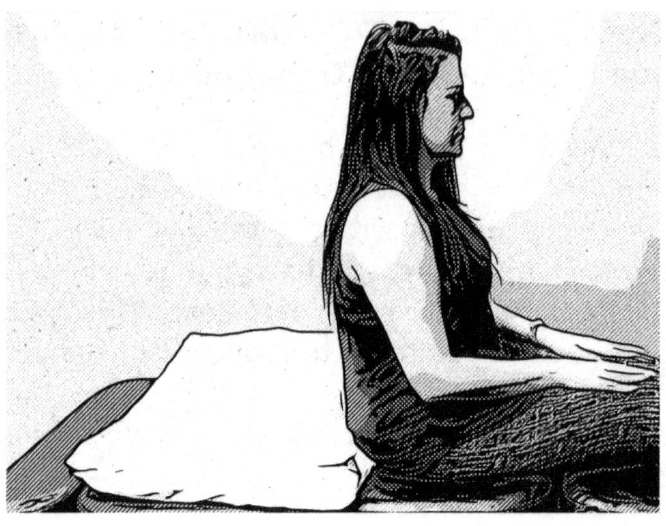

Rotate your neck forty-five degrees to the right. Keeping your eyes open, lie down at a slow to moderate speed (careful, not too fast) so that your shoulders are resting on the pillows and your head is resting lower on the mattress. If you have headaches, mild back or neck issues, do this slower, with assistance.

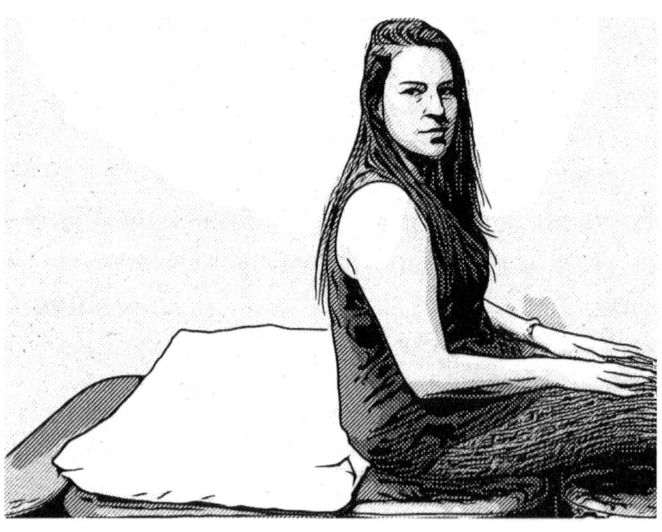

You can also brace your neck with your hand and your back by tightening your tummy muscles. As tolerated, remain in this position for at least thirty seconds. This test is positive for BPPV if your environment visually moves, even when you yourself have stopped moving. If the right-side test is negative, try the left- side test.

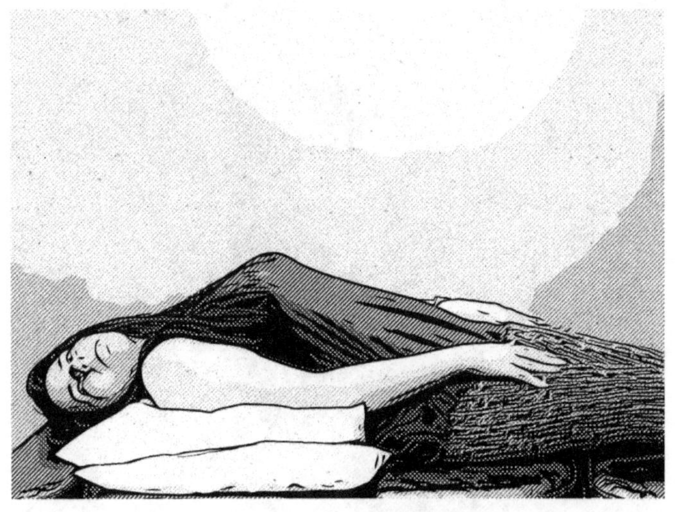

For a video of this, see
https://www.paulgodlewski.com/concussion-dizziness-and-imbalance/

If both tests are negative, you most likely don't have BPPV. However, if you are sure that you do have vertigo, again, consult a vestibular therapist.

Test 2: Anterior Tandem Balance (right-handed individual shown)
Due to the increased risk of injury, I do not recommend this test for anyone sixty-five or older. Instead, I recommend you consult a physiotherapist. If you are in any doubt, for whatever the issue, don't do this test on your own. It's best to check first with your family doctor or a local PT.

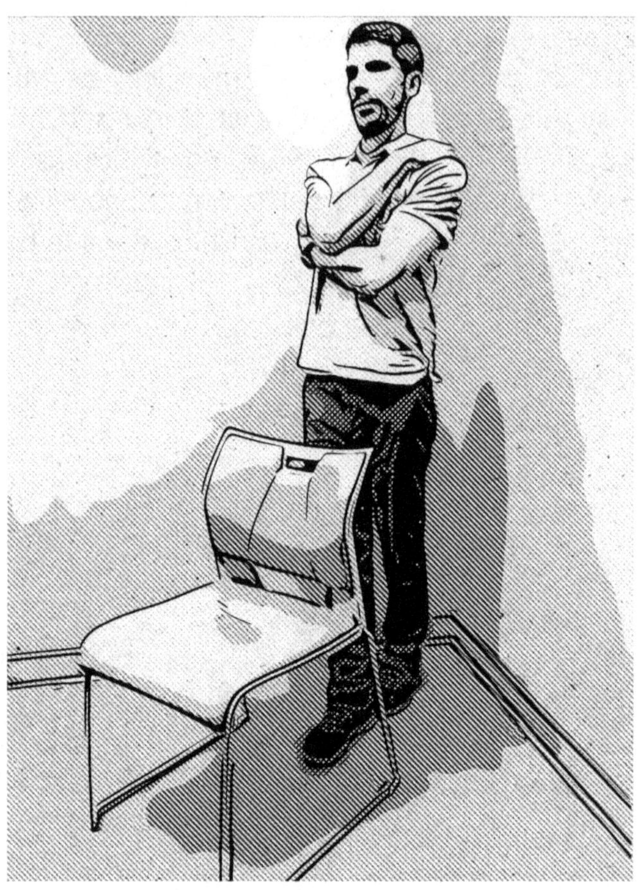

For safety, stand in a corner in your bare feet or in shoes. If you're younger and fitter, cross your arms as shown. Older or less fit individuals should have their hands near the top of the chair (see next). This way, if you lose your balance, you can catch hold of the chair's back. If you're right-handed, place your right foot ahead in line with your left foot (aka tandem stance). Left-handed, the opposite. Initially, do this with your eyes open.

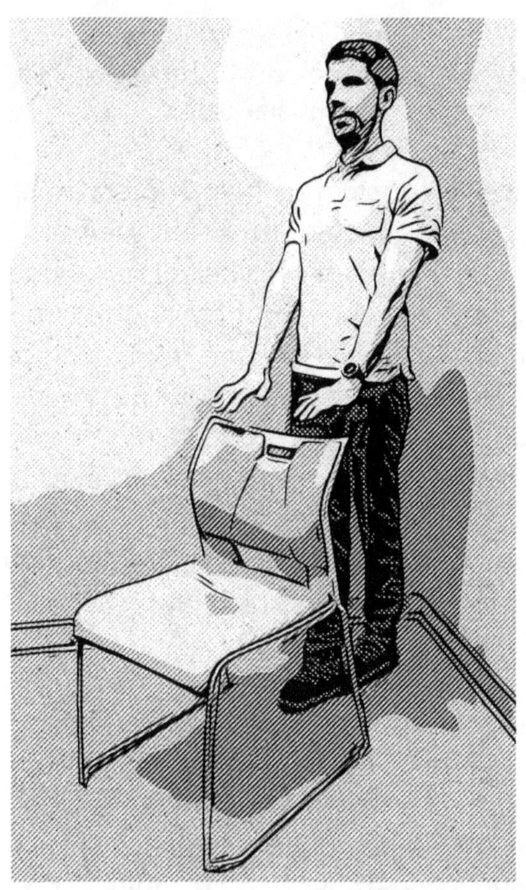

If you can hold this first position relatively easily for approximately thirty seconds, retest with your eyes closed and see how long you can keep your balance. It's best to have someone else time you. Based on your age, the following are norms for the anterior tandem test.11

	Ages 20-49	Ages 50-59	Ages 60-65
Eyes Open	30 sec +/- 3	30 sec +/- 0	29 sec +/- 4
Eyes closed	26 sec +/- 8	21 sec +/- 9	20 sec +/- 11

(For a video of this, see
https://www.paulgodlewski.com/concussion-dizziness-and-
imbalance/)

Your balance is considered *below average for your age range* if you are unable to keep your balance, eyes closed, for the minimum number of seconds shown. For example, if you are between fifty and fifty-nine years of age, you should be able to keep your balance with your eyes closed for at least twelve seconds (i.e., 21seconds - 9 seconds). Your balance is considered *poor for your age* if you can't keep your balance with *eyes open* for the quoted minimum value. For example, if you're aged sixty to sixty-five, you should be able to keep your balance, eyes open, for a minimum of twenty-five seconds (i.e., 29 seconds - 4 seconds).

<u>Test 3</u>: Head Movement Intolerance and Gaze Instability
The following test will inform you if you are having difficulty (or not) tolerating using your vestibular system (specifically the vestibular ocular reflex or VOR) for keeping your gaze stable as you move, or as the world moves around you. Do this test *gently*. Doing it aggressively, or with a big movement of your head, may irritate and even flare up your concussion or neck condition. Without the supervision of a vestibular therapist, do not do this test or its associated exercises in the early days of a concussion (the first three to four weeks). The test is as follows:
- For safety, stand in a corner.
- With your thumb pointing upwards, stretch your hand out in front toward a blank wall.
- Keeping your eyes locked onto your thumb,
- Continuously rotate your head *a smallish amount* from side to side for fifteen to twenty seconds

- Try to change direction about twice per second.
- Older individuals should do this test sitting with their back supported.

(For a video of this, see
https://www.paulgodlewski.com/concussion-dizziness-and-imbalance/)

If you find this worsens some of your symptoms (i.e., feeling off, dizzy, lightheaded, nauseous and/or headachy, but not vertigo, see above), or you are having a hard time keeping up the pace, then this indicates that you may be having problems with your VOR.

Test 4: Motion Sensitivity
This is not something you need to test formally. If during your day-to-day activities (e.g., getting up from bed), your symptoms worsen (i.e., feeling off, dizzy, light-headed, nauseous and/or headachy, but not vertigo, see above), then you know you have motion sensitivity. Your movements need to be on the quicker side to provoke motion sensitivity. Examples of motion sensitivity symptoms include:
- Turning in bed
- Sitting up or lying down in bed
- Bending forward (e.g., to put something in a garbage receptacle)
- Looking upwards (e.g., at an upper shelf)
- Changing directions (e.g., turning in the kitchen)

If you're in doubt, try a couple of the gentler movements, like turning in bed, to self-test. However, like the gaze instability test, this should be done carefully. These too can flare up your concussion or neck if done too aggressively. Without the supervision of a vestibular therapist, do not do this test or its associated exercises in the early days of a concussion (the first three to four weeks). The test is as follows:

6.8 A DIY Approach to Relieving Dizziness and Imbalance

If dizziness, neck pain, and/or headaches persist for more than ten days, the following exercises are recommended. It's important to realize that doing these exercises won't immediately relieve your symptoms. In fact, initially they will likely worsen them a bit. At the same time, use common sense. As a general rule, I tell my patients that none of these exercises should flare their symptoms too much (i.e., greater than two on a scale of ten, where ten out of ten is the worst dizziness that you can imagine).

If you're already feeling dizzy, say at a two out of ten level, then the exercise should not be done to the level that makes it exceed four out of ten (i.e., 2/10 + 2/10). Moreover, I recommend that the exercises should not increase your symptoms for more than ten minutes after you have completed each one. This is especially true for the early days of a concussion. It will take some time for you to overcome these issues. Have patience, be gentle, but be persistent. These exercises work for the vast majority of concussed patients.

Sensory Integration Exercise

There is no specific test that indicates you need to do this exercise. Instead, if you find you are dizzy in your day-to-day activities, this class of exercises is very beneficial regardless. The goal of these exercises is to knit your sensory systems into greater unity, or sensory integration.

If you're going to miss any anti-dizzy exercise, this shouldn't be the one. Its only downside is that it's the most time-consuming of all the exercises I give, though in my experience, it's worth every minute. Consider the time it takes as "you time."

Apart from benefits for your dizziness and disequilibrium, it will also help you with any low mood and/or anxiety because of its mindfulness component. Mindful walking is therefore a "two-for-one deal" exercise. What's not to like about that?

<u>Walking and Looking</u> (aka Mindful Walking)
Find a quiet open space with longer views, such as an outdoor park or quiet residential street. While maintaining your regular walking speed, look forward to the horizon for roughly thirty to sixty seconds (you don't need to be super accurate about this timing). Don't fix your gaze on any one object. Instead, be "open" to the entire horizon. This is called "soft looking." Think of soft looking as the way a wide-angle camera lens would take in the horizon. You're not zooming in on, say, a tree as would a telescopic lens.

Continue walking at a comfortable pace, now at a slow to medium speed. Move both your head and eyes to look at something. Identify this something in your mind and make some sort of comment to yourself (e.g., "hmm, nice red door"). This is a form of "hard looking," like a telescopic lens zooming in on the object. Focus on this thing for only five to ten seconds. Then, for another thirty to sixty seconds, recentre your vision, again soft looking at the horizon. Repeat this process, sometimes looking to the right or left at eye level, sometimes diagonally up or down. Pick things that catch your interest and don't require you to turn your trunk in order to keep them in sight as you walk along.

Rather than a set distance, use a watch or your mobile phone to time your walk. Start by walking, as tolerated, for ten to twenty minutes, four times per week. It's a good idea to alternate this mindful, slower walk with your faster, cardio walk/biking exercise on the other days (see chapter 3). Don't try to save time by combining them. These two exercises are for very different purposes. "As tolerated" means that you should not feel increased symptoms for greater than ten minutes after returning from your walk. If you feel the same or recover within ten minutes, you can increase your walk by two minutes per day. If, for more than ten minutes, you do feel worse than you felt when leaving, reduce your walk by two minutes per day until you find the right amount of time for this initial walking period.

Thereafter, build your walking endurance and tolerance. The goal is eventually to be able to walk sixty minutes a day (thirty to forty minutes for older individuals). As the walk becomes longer, you can break your single walk into two to three walks of shorter duration per day. Older people with poor balance will need to use a cane or walker or be supervised while doing this exercise. In this case, speak to your PT. This exercise only works if you do it regularly and for increasingly longer periods of time. *So, you need to get your walking dosage (i.e., a minimum of four times a week)!*

If the weather is poor, you can do this indoors in the concourse of a shopping mall. But compared to a walk in the open, you may have to reduce the duration of this indoor walk, as it will be much more stimulating for your visual and vestibular systems. You can combine it with doing something else, like going to a corner store to buy milk, as long as you do it mindfully. You can walk with others for companionship, but don't talk during this mindful walk. Don't listen to music or podcasts. You need to concentrate on your walking and looking exercise.

How to Progress This Walking Exercise
Once you have met the goal of sixty minutes straight or cumulatively (thirty to forty minutes for those that are older), you can progress to walking in visually busier and noisy areas. But do so restarting from a shorter period (i.e., restart back at about thirty or forty minutes) and rebuild your tolerance. Examples of this in order of difficulty are as follows:
- Walking in a dappled forest area
- Walking down a narrow alleyway
- Walking indoors in a shopping mall concourse region between the shops
- Walking up and down fluorescent-lit supermarket aisles

Benign Paroxysmal Positional Vertigo (BPPV) Treatment
Do this treatment if Test 1 is positive, either for the left or the right side for real vertigo (see above).

This must be done before proceeding with other exercises; otherwise BPPV will continue to upset your balance system. Theoretically, you can do this yourself, most often with something called the modified Epley's maneuver, but if you have never done this unassisted, it's a bit tricky to know how to interpret the test and to perform the modified Epley's. For this reason, I recommend, at least for the first time, you have a vestibular PT do the assessment and treatment.

Balance Exercises

Not only are balance exercises a good thing in themselves, but as long as you use common sense and take precautions, they are a wonderful way to stimulate neuroplastic recovery in a concussed brain. Optimally, your brain will learn the most if the balance task is neither too hard, nor too easy (i.e., "medium hard" for you to do). Continually adjusting the exercises to be in the medium-hard range will optimize your balance to the best level for you.

Standing Balance Exercises

Do this exercise if Test 2 showed that your balance is below average for your age range. In addition, if during testing your symptoms (e.g., dizziness) increased by no greater than a three on a scale of ten (where ten out of ten is the worst imaginable).

Find a free corner (sometimes hard to do in our furniture and ornament-filled homes). For example, in the corner formed when you close a door. Place one pillow diagonally out from the corner. The pillow should not be too loose or thick. However, it needs to be thick enough so you can't feel the floor. Place a tall, non-rolling chair (e.g., a dining room chair) diagonal to the corner with the back facing inwards. Stand on the pillow facing out from the corner, with your feet apart.

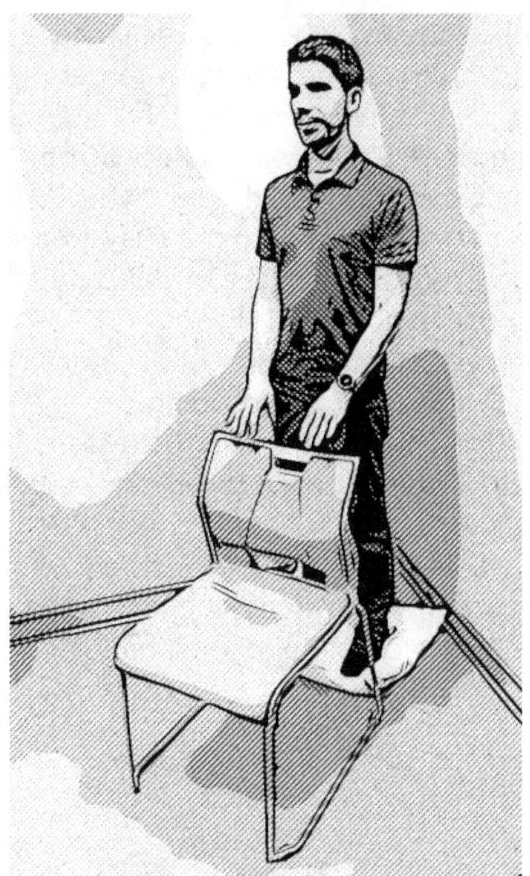

- Stand up straight with your hands just a bit above the back of a chair.
- Start by standing on one pillow with your feet apart. If this is too easy, try two pillows
- Look straight ahead, tighten your tummy and try to hold for up to sixty seconds.

(For a video of this, see
https://www.paulgodlewski.com/concussion-dizziness-and-imbalance/)

Repeat two to three times a day. You will need to do this exercise, along with some progressions, for at least one to two months to see significant improvements.

How and when to progress the static balance exercise: Remember, you're always trying to target medium hard (but never to the point of near fall or actual falls). Progress the exercise if it was too easy from the start or your symptoms have settled (e.g., your dizziness), or because you have improved to the easy-to-medium level of doing the exercise. In order of difficulty, here is how to progress this exercise:

- First bring your feet together until you can balance with your heels and toes touching.
- Now position one foot backwards to stand in a staggered position. This is called semi-tandem standing.
- Gradually bring the foot backwards until you are able to balance with your feet fully in line with one another. This is called tandem standing.

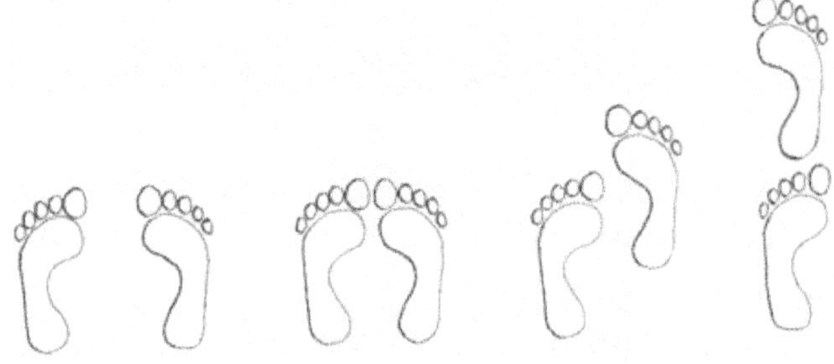

- In the positions that are applicable, switch your feet so you are sometimes doing the exercise right footed, sometimes left footed.

Switch your feet so you are sometimes doing the exercise with your right foot forward, sometimes left. For most people, it will generally be easier when your dominant foot (usually the same side as your dominant hand) is the forward one.

- In this position, stand straight while you slowly and smoothly turn your head.
- The final one is to try to stand on one leg, the hardest being with eyes closed.
- While you do your balance exercise, multitask (e.g., also listening to the radio, reading, etcetera).

Important Note: Not everyone will be able to go to the most advanced level safely. However, any improvement is good.

<u>Day-to-day Practices</u>

Try to use your improving balance in your activities of daily living. For example, while brushing your teeth at the bathroom sink, try standing with your feet closer together, or staggered, and without touching the sink too often. But remember, doing so while performing other tasks is more challenging. Don't jar yourself or fall! Use common sense, and challenge yourself, but only within safe limits.

Gaze Stability Exercises

As discussed earlier in the chapter, you rely on your senses and brain to keep images stable, even though you and/or your environment are moving (e.g., driving).

Do these exercises if Test 3 shows that you have gaze instability.

Start by downloading a free metronome app onto your phone. Alternatively, type the word "metronome" into your internet search field. A metronome is used by musicians to train themselves to play a piece of music at a certain tempo. We will use this device to improve your gaze stability and tolerance to head motions.

As the gaze instability is the result of an injury to the brain itself (e.g., a concussion) or to the neck (e.g., whiplash), you need to be very gentle with these exercises. In the case of concussion, this is because, by rotating your head from side to side, you are, to some degree, reproducing the acceleration and deceleration that caused the initial injury. In the case of whiplash, moving your head too far and too quickly may, if it is too early, irritate the joints that are trying to heal. For severe concussions or whiplash, the initial guidance for these exercises from a vestibular therapist is best.

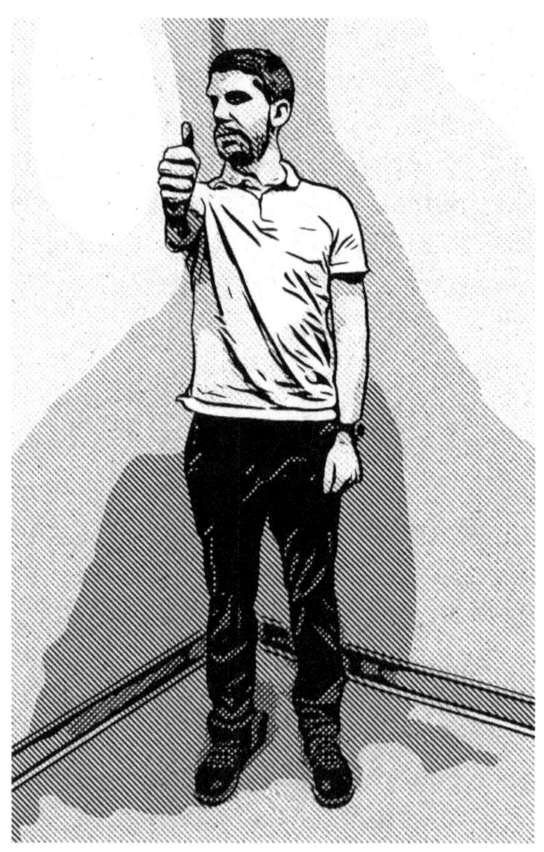

- In this position, stand straight while you slowly and smoothly turn your head.
- Set a metronome initially at sixty beats per minute (bpm).
- Stretch out your arm in front of you with your thumb pointing upwards.
- Keeping your eyes locked onto your thumb, rotate your head side to side a small amount (metaphorically from 11 a.m. to 1 p.m. on a wall clock) in time with the metronome
- Keep doing this for sixty seconds.

- Take a break for a minute or two.
- Again, stretch out your arm in front of you.
- Pitch your head up and down (metaphorically a small amount above and below the center of a wall clock) in time with the metronome for sixty seconds.

For a video of this, see
https://www.paulgodlewski.com/concussion-dizziness-and-imbalance/

Repeat both side to side and up and down two to three times a day. Remember, it's important not to be overly aggressive with this exercise. This should be tolerable. It may cause a worsening of your symptoms, but this worsening should not last longer than sixty minutes or be more than a two or three on a scale of ten in severity. In addition, you must not do this at the expense of the image blurring, or your symptoms. If any of this happens, you will need to slow down the speed (anywhere between thirty to sixty bpm) and/or shorten the duration (anywhere between twenty to sixty seconds). If you continue to have problems, this exercise can be done while seated with your back supported and taking longer breaks (i.e., two to five minutes).

In order of difficulty, here's how to progress this exercise, either because it was too easy from the start or you were able to do it while keeping the rules above:
- Gradually build from being able to do it at 60 bpm for one minute (both side to side and up and down) to 120 bpm for one minute.
- Build from one to two minutes.
- Point your thumb toward a busy background (e.g., a bookshelf or living room area).
- Now do the exercise while you are multitasking by simultaneously completing a balance task. For example, standing on two pillows or with your feet placed in semi-tandem (see the balance exercise above).

<u>Day-to-day Practices</u>
Try to improve your head motion tolerance and gaze stability in your activities of daily living. Remember to use the same rules as above with respect to tolerance (i.e., not too strong an increase in symptoms or for too long). In order of difficulty:
- Have someone drive you for increasing periods of time, first in quiet areas, then in busier ones. In some ways, this is harder than driving. But it is safer to start with.
- Once your doctor has cleared you to drive, drive for increasing periods of time, first in quiet areas, then in busier ones.
- Combine walking with some light jogging (aka interval jogging). As tolerated, lightly jog for one minute, then walk briskly for four minutes. Repeat this interval two to four times. Gradually increase the jogging component until you are jogging for the full interval.

Motion Desensitization (aka Habituation) Exercises

After sustaining an injury, your brain overreacts to motion as a potential threat. You can adjust this back to normal by becoming progressively and *gently* more active and by doing the following motion habituation exercises. For similar reasons to the gaze stability exercises, habituation exercises need to be done gently and, with more severe concussions or whiplashes, are best done initially with the guidance of a vestibular therapist. I generally wait until later in the recovery (six to eight weeks post injury) when the individual is not too symptomatic to initiate these exercises. Again, this is because they are, in part, reproducing the forces of acceleration and deceleration of the original injury. If in doubt, consult your doctor or a vestibular physiotherapist first.

Don't do these exercises until six to eight weeks after your injury. Thereafter, it's worthwhile to do these exercises if you still notice a feeling of dizziness or disequilibrium during day-to-day activities like turning in bed or getting up from bed, or bending appropriately to get something out of a lower cupboard or an upper shelf.

In this exercise, you work on only one movement at a time. The initial movements are designed to be gentle. If a particular movement provokes mild to moderate dizziness or disequilibrium, it tells you that you need to work on that movement until it no longer provokes the symptom, or does so very little. It usually takes some days of doing the exercise to eliminate the symptom reaction. If the symptom provocation is more than a two or three on a scale of ten and/or lasts for more than ten minutes after the movement, then avoid that movement for a week or two and retest. Also, if the movement brings on a sense of movement external to you (aka vertigo), stop the exercise and consult a vestibular therapist. You cannot habituate yourself to BPPV.

Each exercise must be performed with just enough speed to bring on mild to moderate (1-3/10) amounts of dizziness or disequilibrium, but not to cause injury (remember: "more isn't better"). Start with the first exercise in this set. If you don't react to it, you do not need to retest this movement. Instead, move on to the next exercise. On any given day, even if you're not reacting to any of those day's tests/exercises, don't do more than four movements. This is because you may experience a delayed reaction. Best to be a bit conservative and see how you do later that day or the next before proceeding to a more advanced test/exercise.

If you're having neck or back issues, consult your GP or physiotherapist before engaging in these exercises. This is especially true for exercises such as sitting up or lying back relatively quickly. Once cleared, if your neck is irritated, you may need to brace your neck by supporting it with your hand. In general, before doing any movement, it's good practice to tighten your tummy muscles without holding your breath to protect your back (aka bracing your back with core muscles).

Repeat each exercise three times in a row, with a bit of a break between each repetition. Do the exercise one to two times a day. By doing these exercises, you will gradually, movement by movement, lessen and eventually eliminate your motion sensitivity.

The motions in order of difficulty are as follows:

- Lying on your back with your head on a pillow and your knees bent, tighten your tummy muscles and quickly roll like a log to your RIGHT side. Wait for symptoms to pass, then a bit longer before proceeding to the next repetition. Once this no longer bothers you, move on to turning to your LEFT side.
- Lying on your back with your legs straight and your head on a pillow, tighten your tummy muscles and quickly sit up (brace your neck if needed). Wait for symptoms to pass, then a bit longer before proceeding to the next repetition.
- Sitting on the bed with your legs outstretched, tighten your tummy muscles and drop back (brace your neck if needed) so that your head is on a pillow. Do not throw yourself back, but perform this at a mild to moderate speed so your head **does not strike** the pillow hard. Wait for symptoms to pass, then a bit longer before proceeding to the next repetition.
- Sit in a chair with your knees apart. Tighten your tummy muscles and quickly tip your head toward your RIGHT knee. **Do not strike** your head on your knee. Wait for symptoms to pass, then a bit longer before proceeding to the next repetition. Once this no longer bothers you, move on to doing this toward the LEFT knee.
- Sit in a chair with your knees apart and your head tipped to your RIGHT knee. Tighten your tummy muscles and quickly sit upright (brace your neck if needed), so you're now facing forward. Wait for symptoms to pass, then a bit longer before proceeding to the next repetition. Once this no longer bothers you, move on to doing this coming up from the LEFT knee.

For a video of this, see
https://www.paulgodlewski.com/concussion-dizziness-and-imbalance/

<u>Day-to-Day Practices</u>
Most of these exercises are things you do in your day-to-day practice. Therefore, it is not necessary to prescribe more.

6.9 When Not to Go It Alone

Apart from cautions and contraindication noted in section 6.3 about red flags, there are a number of other reasons you may not want to go it alone:

- If the thought of testing or doing these exercises by yourself is just too much for you
- If you know in your heart of hearts that you're not likely to continue doing the exercise without the assistance or nudge from a PT
- If you need to use a walking aid, such as a cane or a walker

In these cases, I recommend you consult a good vestibular physiotherapist (PT). There are a number of ways a specially trained vestibular and concussion physiotherapist can help you beyond what you can do on your own, such as providing more advanced exercises (e.g., dynamic balance exercise walking). In addition, they can assess the need for neck proprioception training, substitution exercises, and the use of special orthotics, weighted blankets, and/or compression vests.

References

1. Olesen, J. et al. 2018. "The International Classification of Headache Disorders, 3rd edition." *Cephalalgia*, 38, no. 1, 1–211. https://doi.org/10.1177/0333102417738202

2. Szczupak, M. et al. 2016. "Posttraumatic dizziness and vertigo." in *Handbook of Clinical Neurology - Neuro-Otology.* Vol. 137 Chapter 21. Editors Furman J.M. and Lempert, T. 2016. Oxford, United Kingdom. Elsevier.

3. Davies, R. and Luxon, L. 1995. "Dizziness Following Head Injury: A Neuro-Otological Study." *J. Neurol* 242, no. 4 (April), 222–230. https://doi.org/10.1007/BF00919595

4. Crampton A., et al. 2021 "Vestibular-Ocular Reflex Dysfunction Following Mild Traumatic Brain Injury: A Narrative Review." *Neurochirurgie* 67, no. 3 (May), 231–237. https://doi.org/10.1016/j.neuchi.2021.01.002

5. Chamelian L. and Feinstein A. 2004. "Outcome after Mild to Moderate Traumatic Brain Injury: The Role of Dizziness." *Arch Phys Med Rehabil.* 85, no. 10 (Oct), 1662–6. https://www.archives-pmr.org/article/S0003-9993(04)00307-7/fulltext

6. Womble, M. et al. 2021. "Risk Factors for Vestibular and Oculomotor Outcomes After Sport-Related Concussion." *Clin J Sport Med.* 31, no 4 (Jul) e193-e199. https://doi.org/10.1097/JSM.0000000000000761

7. Mucha, A. et al. 2018. "Vestibular dysfunction and concussion." in *Handbook of Clinical Neurology - Neuro-Otology.* Vol. 158 Chapter 14, Editors Hainline, B. Stern, R.A. Oxford, United Kingdom, Elsevier.

8. Schneider K.J., et al. 2014. "Cervicovestibular Rehabilitation in Sport-Related Concussion: A Randomised Controlled Trial." *Br J Sports Med* 48, no. 17 (Sep), 1294–1298. https://doi.org/10.1136/bjsports-2013-093267

9. Marshall, C.M. et al. 2015 "The Role of the Cervical Spine in Post-Concussion Syndrome." *Phys Sportsmed* 43 no. 3 (Jul), *274–284. https://doi.org/10.1080/00913847.2015.1064301*

10. Reiley A. L. et al. 2017. "How to Diagnose Cervicogenic Dizziness." *Archives of Physiotherapy* 7 no 12, 1-12. https://doi.org/10.1186/s40945-017-0040-x

11. El-Kashlan H.K., et al. (1998). Evaluation of clinical measures of equilibrium. *Laryngoscope 108* (3) 311-319. https://doi.org/10.1097/00005537-199803000-00002

Chapter 7

Vision Issues

"The eye sees only what the mind is prepared to comprehend." Robertson Davies

Cheat Sheet

7.1 How Evelyn Overcame Vision Problems

Evelyn sustained a concussion from falling on her patio. The concussion led to significant problems with her vision and greatly contributed to her headaches and dizziness, which slowed her recovery.

7. 2 But My Ophthalmologist/Optometrist Says My Eyes Are Normal!

This section explains how, following a concussion, your eyes can still be technically "normal" while you continue having significant and prolonged issues with your vision.

7.3 Parts of Your Vision, You Didn't Even Know You Had

I discuss the different capacities of your visual system. When everything is working well, these components effortlessly and seamlessly give you something we call vision.

7.4 What Is Neuro-Optometry?

Neuro-optometry's focus is the same as regular optometry but, in addition, treats visual dysfunction associated with brain injury (e.g., concussion).

7.5 Deep Dive: Neuro-Optometrists See Vision as a Two-Part Harmony

Read this if you would like to learn more than one theory about how your vision works, the emerging but still early evidence for vision therapy, and who should be providing it.

7.6 Tests to See if a DIY Approach Will Likely Help *Some* Vision Functional Issues

Two very important questions you need to ask yourself *before* you embark on a DIY approach to vision treatments.

7.7 A DIY Approach to Help *Some* Vision Functional Issues

If indicated by the tests above, I give you a selection of exercises you can do to help your vision improve via neuroplastic recovery.

7.8 When Not to Go It Alone

Reasons why you should not take a DIY approach to vision exercising.

7.1 How Evelyn Overcame Vision Problems

Being retired, Evelyn was able to do all the things she loved best, like puttering midweek in the garden with her husband. Even two years on from her retirement, it still made her feel like she was playing "hooky" from work. Unfortunately, that thought was one of the last she could later recall from the time just before her accident. As she walked across the uneven flagstones of their patio, her husband observed her catch her foot and fall. On her way down, he saw her take a glancing blow to the back of her head on a patio table before striking her head once more on the ground.

She lost consciousness and regained it only later in the ambulance. At the hospital, she couldn't remember the event at all. She told the emergency doctor she was feeling dizzy and had difficulty focusing, as well as double vision. All the tests at emergency, including a CT scan, came back as normal. She was diagnosed with a concussion and released to the care of her family doctor. Later, examinations by an ophthalmologist and an otolaryngologist (ENT) found no problems structurally with either her eyes or her ears, respectively.

When her symptoms had settled a bit, her family doctor referred her to a sports doctor, as well as a physiotherapist experienced in vestibular rehabilitation therapy (VRT). Evelyn told the VRT PT that she was still experiencing constant dizziness. Her blurred vision and double vision were intermittent, but in addition, she now had great difficulty concentrating, fogginess, motion sickness, poor balance, and headaches. On examining her, the physiotherapist observed that her symptoms seemed most related to significant issues involving both her balance and vision systems (aka vestibular oculomotor dysfunction). The VRT therapist referred her to a neuro-optometrist colleague.

Her team consisted of medical management by a sports physician, concussion rehabilitation management and vestibular treatment by her physiotherapist, and vision therapy from a neuro-optometrist (including use of prism glasses). It took her fourteen months to fully return to feeling like her pre-accident self. Given the complexity of her issues, a DIY approach would not have been sufficient to get her there.

7.2 But My Ophthalmologist/Optometrist Says My Eyes Are Normal!

Well good, you did exactly the right thing by having your eyes checked out. This is because a concussion can also injure your eye or optic nerve. The ophthalmologist or optometrist will check all your eye structures for injury (aka visual structural dysfunction): cornea, iris, lenses, retina, and optic nerve. They will determine visual acuity and your peripheral vision capacity. They may also check your eye pressure. The good news is that, in the vast majority of cases, your eyes will be completely uninjured.

So, if everything is normal, why do your eyes hurt? Why do you have difficulty concentrating on what you are looking at? And why do you get headaches, especially when you try to read? The ophthalmologist or optometrist finding no problems with these structures unfortunately does not rule out that you may have problems functionally with your vision (aka vision dysfunction). Visual functional issues occur when your brain has difficulty moving your eyes around as efficiently as normal (aka oculomotor problems).

Most non-vision professionals think vision is just your ability to read an eye chart (aka the Snellen Chart). Such a chart helps the eye care professional find how clearly you can see at a certain distance. This is known as your acuity. But this is just one of the many things your eyes do to give you what we call sight.

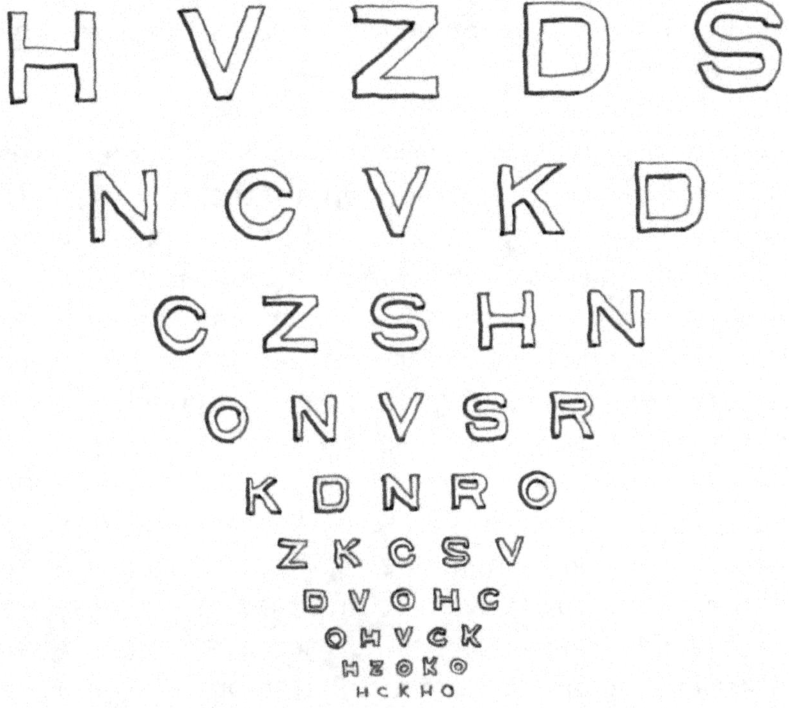

In addition to what your eyes do, your brain plays the important role of bringing meaning out of all the information coming from your eyes. Seeing is not just about your eyes' internal health and visual acuity. Vision problems can occur anywhere from the level of the eyes, all the way up to the nerve tracks in the brain, and finally to any of the multiple regions in your brain that interpret what you are seeing. Potentially having cellular injuries, concussions can affect any or all the parts that contribute to your ability to see.

7.3 Parts of Your Vision, You Didn't Even Know You Had

...but you were secretly waiting for someone to tell you about. Okay, maybe not, but with a bit of patience, you'll understand what's going on (or not, as the case may be) with your vision.

Vision is best thought of as a series of skill steps. From the very simplest, lowest step to the highest, most complex step, they work together so smoothly and seamlessly that you don't even realize it. Each skill step relies on the simpler skills below it having done their job properly. In addition, the brain's preconceptions of what you are seeing have a significant—and arguably bigger—impact on what you end up seeing. For example, you already know what a chair looks like. Coming upon a chair, all your brain has to do is slightly tweak the chair it already has in its mind's eye. These visual skill steps, starting at the lowest, can be arranged as: visual acuity, visual field, fixating/unfixating, accommodation, global attention, versions, vergence, stereopsis, and visual perception. Rather than define each of these, I'm going to present you with a story to show you how all these skills knit together to give you this amazing ability called vision.

You are at a party. Out of the corner of your eye (the far visual field) you see a vertical object. Turning your head and focusing in on it (visual acuity), you see it's an object with a round bit at the top, a shape in the middle, and two slender, somewhat separated, rectangles on the ground. It's moving toward you, so you need to keep your eyes locked onto it (visual fixation) and continually adjust your eyes to keep it in focus (visual accommodation).

You also need to concentrate (global attention), as there are so many other distracting things going on at this party: other sights, conversations, not to mention that absolutely delicious smell coming from the kitchen. *No, you say to yourself, I'll check all that out later!*

Good thing you paid attention, because this thing has suddenly changed direction. Your eyes need to follow it toward another something (version—smooth pursuit) that sort of resembles it but is not quite the same shape. You are just starting to feel disappointed (not sure why yet?) when you note it's back on track and coming toward you. [Now, don't be impatient, this is only going to take another few milliseconds.]

It's getting closer now, so much so that you have to bring your eyes closer together (convergence) to stop the object from doubling. So close, in fact, you are picking up a wonderful scent. *Concentrate* (global attention)! As your two eyes are seeing it from slightly different angles, you now realize (via stereopsis) it's a series of oh-so-nice, frankly wow, volumes! Okay, it really has your full attention now. *Hold on. What's it holding?* You shift your eyes quickly down (version—saccade) and focus in (visual acuity). Uh-oh, it's a gun! (visual perception). *And this was going so well!* (sigh)

Obviously, this does not happen one step at a time but all at once and very quickly. Even when you have had a concussion, it will continue to work in this way. But often a concussion will make it much more effortful and symptom-provoking to perform all these little visual actions that are a normal part of everyone's day (well all except, hopefully, the gun!).

7.4 What Is Neuro-Optometry?

Both optometry and ophthalmology focus on promoting eye health, remediating pathology of the structures of the eye (e.g., the lens, retina, optic nerve, etcetera), and providing equipment such as glasses or contact lenses to overcome visual limitation (e.g., astigmatism). In addition, as medical eye doctors, ophthalmologists can perform eye surgery.

Neuro-optometry is a specialized branch of optometry. Its goals are the same as regular optometry, but in addition, they use the principles of neuroplasticity to overcome the brain's problems in visual function. Neuro-optometric treatment relies on the brain's ability to observe patterns and correct its own faults through neuroplastic change (see chapter 2). To encourage neuroplastic recovery, the patient works on progressively harder vision exercises, plus or minus visual aids (e.g., prism glasses, bi-nasal occlusion, and tints).[1] They also work on more complex visual processing and perceptual deficits such as manifesting as figure-ground disturbances, sensory integration, and delay issues, etcetera. These are too complex to explain in a DIY book.

7.5 Deep Dive: Neuro-Optometrists See Vision as a Two-Part Harmony

I am going to start this Deep Dive by introducing you to a theory that has emerged from neuro-optometry. In order to negotiate your environment, your brain takes information from multiple sources, including the eyes and other senses around your body. The brain then uses all this information to keep you safe, plan, make decisions, control movement, etcetera. Working with patients with a wide variety of neurological conditions, Dr. Padula, a well-respected US doctor of optometry, developed a theory that vision is not just one thing (unimodal), but in fact has two parts (bimodal).[2] Normally they work together so well and seamlessly that you are unaware that there are two major parts: the ambient and focal systems.

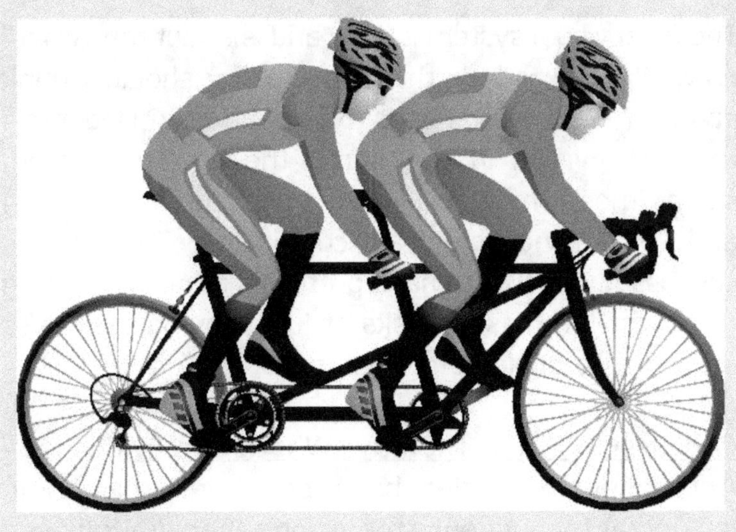

A brief story will help to show how these parts work together. Lucky you, you're reading a guidebook while walking in some lovely European city. In the background, the ambient system works with many other senses to keep your balance and inform you about where you are and what you need to do to avoid other people and obstacles. It also helps your eyes move from one word to the next in the guidebook.

Meanwhile your focal system is left to concentrate on the content of the book, the maps, and text so you can decide where you are going. The ambient visual system is thought to be very fast but relatively poor in detail (i.e., not the "what" of a situation). It is more concerned about the "where and when," particularly the future. It's also key to knowing how to move your eyes.

The focal visual system is slow and is about the "what" now. What exactly is this thing? What should I think about it? What really needs to be done now? Under this theory of vision in two parts, the ambient system seems most prone to trouble in concussion (mTBIs) and other neurological conditions. This leads concussed patients to have problems most often doing the lower-level visual tasks of just moving their eyes around (aka oculomotor dysfunction).

<u>Concussion Vision Therapy: What's the Evidence</u>?
A number of studies have been very helpful in looking at the evidence for vision rehabilitation used

for concussions (mTBI). Hunt and colleagues looked at the assessment of visual dysfunction. They found preliminary evidence that clinical measurements of saccades, smooth pursuit, and vergence were useful in detecting change in cases of concussion (mTBI).[3] Berger and colleagues, in their systematic review of occupational therapist's vision treatment, found variability in the effectiveness of treatments based on which interventions were employed.[4]

Simpson and colleagues' review focused only on research aimed at basic visual skills (i.e., oculomotor control and acuity). They winnowed down over 2,500 articles to just twenty-two studies. Ninety-five percent of the studies reported at least one improvement in basic vision skills and associated reductions in visually related symptoms. Only one study, related to the use of hyperbaric oxygen to improve basic vision skills, found no improvement. A number of limitations were identified by the authors of this meta study: 77 percent of the studies had forty or fewer participants, symptom duration varied from one week to thirty years, none of the studies employed multidisciplinary interventions, and children, youth (twelve to eighteen), and older individuals were poorly represented. [5]

While literature surveys like this are very useful for clinicians, they do have limitations intrinsic to their nature. The studies reviewed were very different from one another, both in design and quality. For example, in the twenty-two studies reviewed by Simpson and Hunt, the number of treatments reported varied widely. When defined, in-lab treatments (training a wide variety of skills) varied from thirty-six minutes to forty-five minutes per session. The number of sessions varied from six to sixteen sessions. Duration of treatments lasted from two weeks to eight months. Only one study reported a protocol of fifteen minutes per day, five days a week of home exercises. A number of other studies reported home exercise but did not specify the frequency.[5]

Given the limitations above, it becomes necessary to mine deeper down to the individual study level. Five studies by Thiagarajan and Ciuffreda are worthy of more detailed discussion.[6-10] The first four articles all used the same crossover and sham design (single blind) and twelve participants. To avoid time-related recovery, all participants had had their visual disability for at least one year. Only lab-based oculomotor training (OMT) was employed. This OMT comprised forty-five-minute sessions, two times per week, over six weeks (total nine hours). The authors reported a great majority of the basic vision skills were improved to a significant level. These included: reading speed, saccadic movement accuracy, rhythmicity, convergence/divergence speed, accommodation capacity, and decreased fixation errors. In addition, reading comfort and subjective visual attention were significantly enhanced. By the end of the training regime, some of the thirteen parameters returned to normal, others were improved to a significant level, and some showed a trend toward improvement. During the crossover sham training period, no improvements occurred in any of these parameters. [6-9] A fifth study investigated how gains made by the above participants persisted following treatment.

In this study, eight of the twelve individuals were retested at the three- and six-month point following training. No OMT was done between these follow-up periods. It was reported that eight of the thirteen parameters were either maintained or continued to improve upon retesting. The authors hypothesized that, with a doubling of the training period, more parameters would be returned to normal or to a significant level.[10]

Notwithstanding the valid criticisms regarding number of participants, etcetera, these five studies constitute good preliminary evidence for the effectiveness of vision therapy. Clinicians working with these patients can now have more confidence that, properly done, vision therapy can be helpful. In addition, given the conservative, low-risk nature of these therapies, it's not practical to wait until all the evidence is ironclad before trying to help patients with vision therapy. Nevertheless, further research is much needed to raise this confidence level. As always with rehab treatments, the questions of when, where, and frequency also require much, much more research. This seems especially important in the case of vision therapy, as appointments are expensive, not covered by public health systems, and are rarely covered by the patient's extended health insurance. It's known that neuroplastic change (needed in the recovery of all TBIs) takes time. The goal of treatment therefore should be to accelerate and improve this natural neuroplastic recovery.

Concussion Vision Treatment – Who Should Be Providing It?

In my opinion, having a neuro-optometrist on a concussed patient's team is valuable, arguably indispensable, for moderate to severe concussions. Neuro-optometrists possess the educational base and specialized knowledge of vision assessments from structural, pathological, and functional issues. They have the expertise to customize oculomotor training (OMT) to the individual's needs and the ability to prescribe, if needed, medication and assistive equipment (e.g., yoked prism glasses). With respect to resource limitations specifically for vision therapy (which is often quite expensive), I recommend the following to my patients:

- If the individual has good financial resources/insurance coverage and sufficient energy, they should optimally consult the best professional for a given issue (e.g., a neuro-optometrist for vision issues). Oftentimes, the proper neuro-optometric glasses prescription (microprisms, specialized tints, etcetera) can make a tremendous difference quickly, as well as enhance other treatments and therapies.

> • If their resources, both financial and/or energy-wise, are more limited, it is important that the patient try to do as much as they can safely on their own. Thereafter, they can supplement their own efforts by consulting a neuro-optometrist.

7.6 Tests to See if a DIY Approach Is Likely to Help *Some* Vision Functional Issues

Before you test yourself to see if a DIY approach could be helpful, there are two very important questions to ask.

<u>Question 1</u>: Should you consult an ophthalmologist or see an optometrist?

Yes. Only when you have been given the all-clear for your eyes should you even consider whether to attempt a DIY approach, in whole or in part, and/or seek professional help from a neuro-optometrist.

<u>Question 2</u>: How do you know if visual functional dysfunctions are part of your concussion?

To help you answer this, ask yourself the following supplementary questions. These answers are only relevant if this is something new for you following your concussion:

• Do I tend to get headaches/migraines when using my eyes more?

• Do I tend to get dizzy or nauseous when using my eyes more?

- Do I tend to feel foggier when using my eyes more?

- When reading, do I get discomfort in and around my eyes or in my head?

- Does reading screens bother me more than reading the printed page?

- Do I have difficulty comprehending what I am reading?

- Do I have difficulty keeping my attention on what I read?

- Does watching moving objects increase my symptoms?

- Does watching moving objects make stationary objects appear to move?

- Do I seem to bump into things above me, like a cupboard shelf?

- Do I seem to bump into things to one side of me, like a doorframe?

The more of these questions you answer, "yes" to, the more likely you *may* have some visual dysfunction.

Though this quiz is a good first step, it does not in itself provide enough information to determine if you actual have concussion-related visual functional dysfunctions. That is because many of these problems can come from other concussion-related issues, for example, from an inner ear processing problem (see chapter 6).

To better determine if you are having concussion-related visual functional dysfunctions, try the following five visual tests. Pay attention to how each of these tests makes you feel. See if any of them bring on, or worsen, your:

- headache/head pressure;
- eye discomfort/pressure;
- dizziness;
- nausea; and/or
- fogginess.

The tests might bring on other symptoms, but these are the main ones. Always give yourself time to somewhat recover *before* trying the next test. This is because the symptoms can be delayed and/or build up. Taking more time between the tests will give you a better idea of whether you have a problem, and in what area.

<u>Test 1</u>: Smooth Pursuit
- Sit with your back supported, your arm stretched out in front of you and your thumb pointing up to the ceiling.
- With your eyes alone, watch your thumb move side to side at a moderate speed horizontally from the right to the left across your body and back, twice.
- There and back counts as once.
- Make sure to keep your head still while you do this.

How much are your symptoms changed by this test?
None □ (0/5) Mildly □ (1/5) Mildly to moderately □ (2/5)
    Moderately to severely □ (3/5) Severely □ (4-5/5)

<u>Test 2</u>: Horizontal Saccadic Eye Movements
- Between two objects that are about sixty to ninety centimeters apart and at the same height.

- Keeping your head still, move your eyes horizontally back and forth from one object to the other ten times.
- There and back counts as one.
- Do this as quickly as you can, but without blurring.

How much are your symptoms changed by this test?
None □ (0/5) Mildly □ (1/5) Mildly to moderately □ (2/5) Moderately to severely □ (3/5) Severely □ (4-5/5)

Test 3: Vertical Saccadic Eye Movements
- Between two objects that are in a vertical line and about sixty centimeters apart.
- While keeping your head still, move your eyes up and down ten times.
- There and back counts as one.
- Do this as quickly as you can without blurring.

How much are your symptoms changed by this test?
None □ (0/5) Mildly □ (1/5) Mildly to moderately □ (2/5) Moderately to severely □ (3/5) Severely □ (4-5/5)

Test 4: Near-Far Accommodation
- Sit about 245 centimeters (or 8') away from a closed door.
- Stretch out your arm towards the centre of the door with your thumb up.
- Keeping your head still, move your eyes back and forth quickly 10 times between your thumb and the doorknob.
- But ensure your eyes come into focus each time.

How much are your symptoms changed by this test?
None □ (0/5) Mildly □ (1/5) Mildly to moderately □ (2/5) Moderately to severely □ (3/5) Severely □ (4-5/5)

<u>Test 5</u>: Convergence
- While seated, hold a pen at arm's length, level with your nose and pointing toward the ceiling.
- At a slow to medium speed, bring the end of the pen toward your nose at the same time try visually to keep the pen from doubling.
- Repeat this movement three times in total.
- In combination, notice how these movements make you feel.
- Now repeat the test.
- If and when the pen doubles for you, stop and have someone measure from the tip of your nose to the pen.
- The pen will blur, but only where the pen doubles should be noted.

How much are your symptoms changed by this test?
None □ (0/5) Mildly □ (1/5) Mildly to moderately □ (2/5) Moderately to severely □ (3/5) Severely □ (4-5/5)

Does your thumb <u>double</u> or become a shadow of itself before it is 10-15 cm from your nose? Yes □ No □

For a video of this, see
https://www.paulgodlewski.com/concussion-vision-issues/

If any of these tests give you symptoms at the four or five level on a scale of five, or if doubles a distance greater than 15 cm from you nose, it's best to consult a neuro-optometrist.

7.7 A DIY Approach to *Some* Visual Functional Dysfunctions

If you want to encourage neuroplastic recovery, regular and frequent repetition is an absolute must! There is unfortunately *"no free lunch"* when it comes to encouraging neuroplasticity.

Version - Smooth Pursuit Exercises

Do this exercise if Test 1 brings on only a mild or mild-to-moderate increase in your symptoms.

Usually, this exercise is done standing. But if your balance is poor or this makes you dizzy, start doing it while seated. Wear the appropriate glasses, if needed. The background in front of you should be relatively plain (e.g., a neutrally painted wall). Make sure to hold your head still and keep a good, elongated standing/sitting posture (i.e., as if you are a puppet and someone has pulled your centre string).

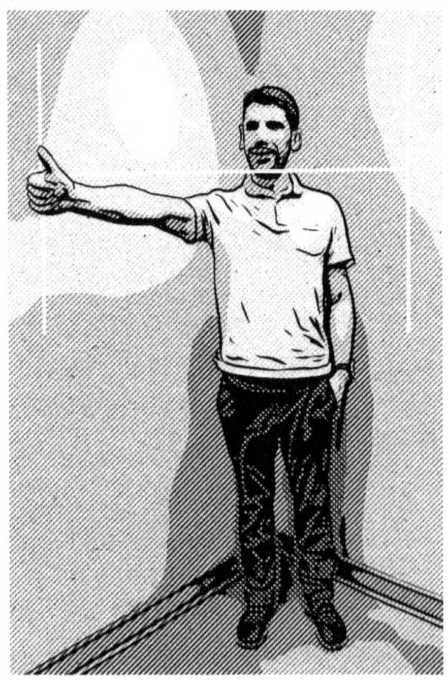

- Stretch out your arm with your thumb pointing to the ceiling.
- Keeping you head still, as shown, follow your thumb with your eyes, while it draws a slow, wide and large H pattern.

For a video of this, see
https://www.paulgodlewski.com/concussion-vision-issues

Do all these movements as slowly as you need to, in order to keep your eyes on your thumb and your thumb in focus. By concentrating on your thumb for the whole time, you are also building your global attention stamina.

Build, as tolerated, from being able to do this for thirty seconds to two minutes per session, two to three times per day. (If evenings are hard on you, just do the exercises earlier two times per day).

If this exercise brings on a lot of symptoms or it is very difficult to do, perform it lying flat on your back with one arm stretched up to the ceiling. If you're still too symptomatic or you can't do the exercise properly, do it with one eye covered by a towel, again lying flat on your back with your arm stretched up to the ceiling.

<u>Here is how to progress this exercise</u>:

- When you are able, move your thumb faster, but make sure you keep your eyes focused on your thumb throughout, and keep your head as still as you can.

- Change the *H* pattern to an infinity triangular pattern with diagonal movements. Again, slower is easier than faster.

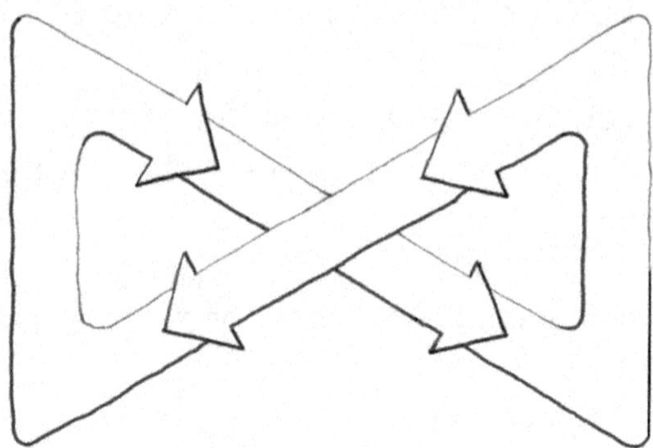

- Change the infinity triangular to a clockwise pattern.

- Then do it as a counterclockwise spiral pattern.

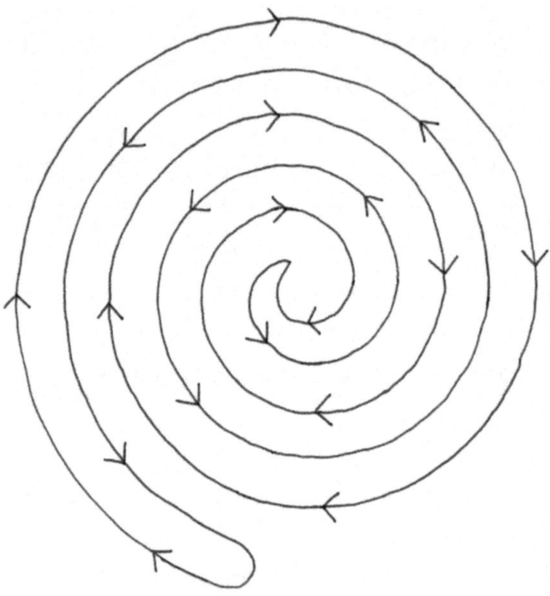

- Now go back to following you thumb as it does a relatively slow *H* pattern. But do it with your head turned comfortably to the right, then with your head turned to the left.

- As previously shown, you can also progress this by doing it faster and /or with the other patterns. The next progression is to do this exercise while practicing your balance (in this case with your feet in the semi-tandem position). Make sure you do this in a corner and have a chair back in front of you so you can hold onto it if you start to lose your balance. You do not want to jar yourself by falling!

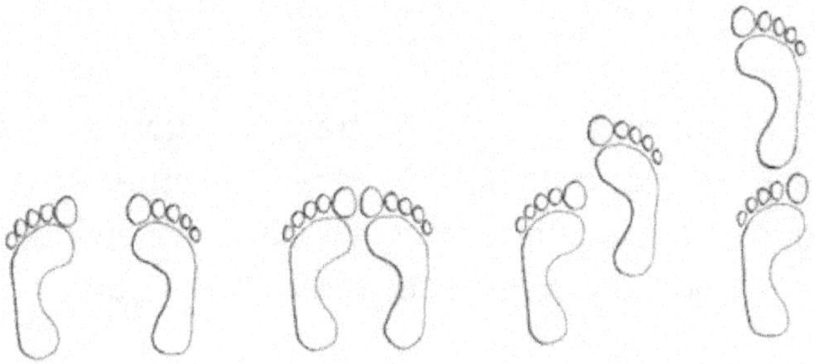

- Do these exercises while practicing your balance, and with your head turned one way or the other. First do them moving your head slowly, then faster and finally incorporating the different patterns previously shown.
- Do the exercise in front of a demanding visual background (e.g., busy wallpaper).
- Do the exercise with an added noise distraction (e.g., while listening to some harmonious music or a conversation on the radio/TV).

<u>Day-to-Day Practices</u> (in order of difficulty)
Use your imagination. The following is just a small sample using this skill. Make sure to hold your head still and keep a good, elongated standing/sitting posture.
- Watch something moving slowly by you (e.g., a baby crawling by).
- Watch a person walking across your field of vision.

- Watch someone climbing a ladder.
- From the side, watch someone go up an escalator or an outside staircase.
- Watch a car moving slowly across your field of vision.
- Watch a bus or train go by faster.
- Follow a butterfly or moth slowly and randomly fluttering around.
- Follow a bird moving more quickly and randomly.
- Watch something like a roller coaster do a loop-to-loop.

You can make all these things harder if you do them for progressively longer times, stand rather than sit, randomly change the target you are following, safely challenge your balance (see above), and add noise or brighter light to the task.

Version – Saccadic Eye Motion Exercises

Do this exercise if Test 2 and/or Test 3 bring(s) on only a mild or mild-to-moderate increase in your symptoms. Usually, this exercise is done standing. But if your balance is poor or this makes you dizzy, start doing it while seated. Wear your glasses, if needed. Make sure to hold your head still and keep a good, elongated standing/sitting posture. Start by copying this basic chart of "Letters and Numbers."

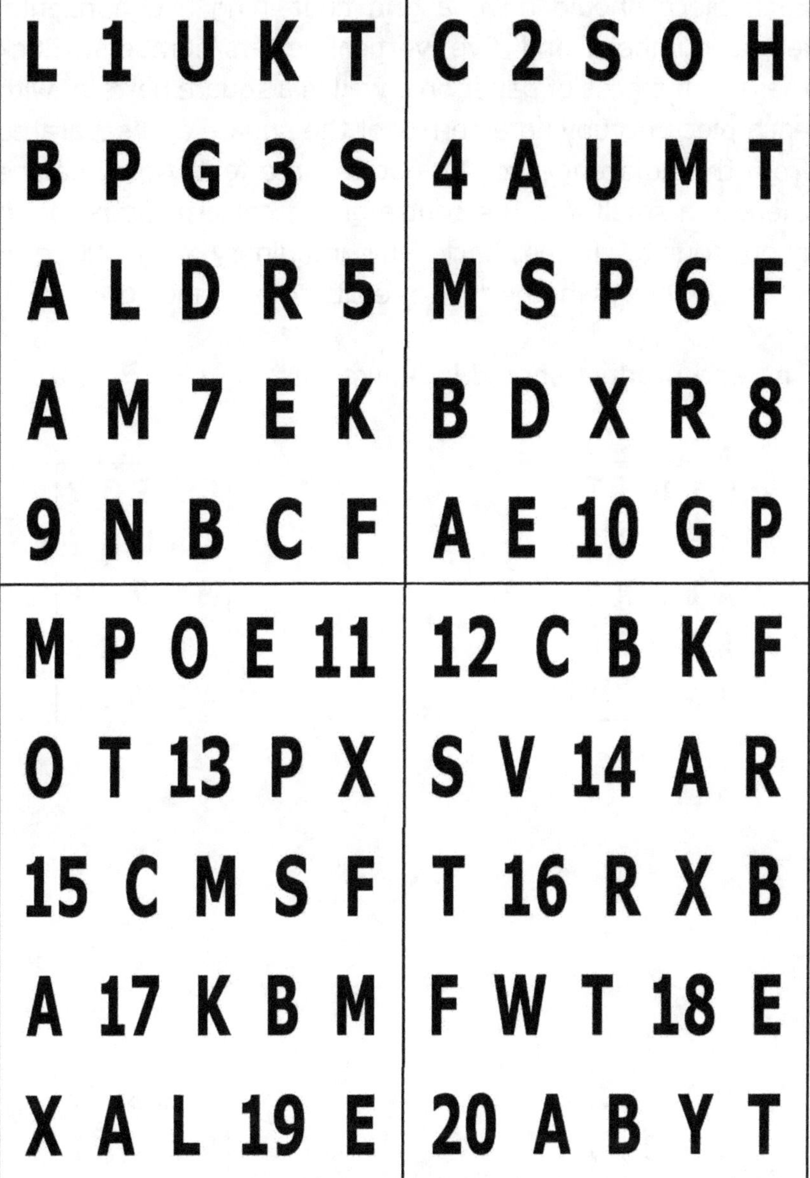

See Appendix G and
https://www.paulgodlewski.com/concussion-exercise-tools-and-appendices/

Cut along the lines to give you four equally sized pieces.

Each piece should have a grid containing five horizontal letters/numbers and five vertical letters/numbers. Stick these four pieces of paper on a wall in a square pattern, with each piece occupying a corner of the square and separated from the adjacent piece by about three feet. Now imagine there is a small *X* in the centre of the pattern. Stand or sit about four to six feet back. This imaginary *X* should be at your eye level, whether you are sitting or standing.

The end product should look like this:

<table>
<tr><td>

L	1	U	K	T
B	P	G	3	S
A	L	D	R	5
A	M	7	E	K
9	N	B	C	F

</td><td>

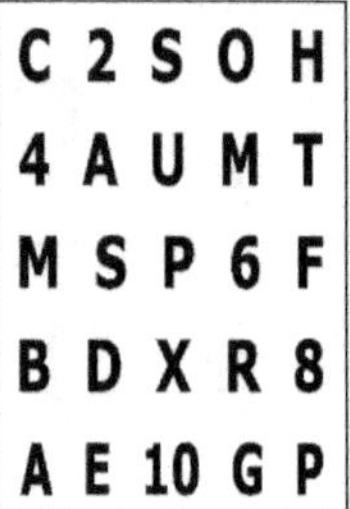

C	2	S	O	H
4	A	U	M	T
M	S	P	6	F
B	D	X	R	8
A	E	10	G	P

</td></tr>
</table>

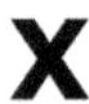

<table>
<tr><td>

M	P	O	E	11
O	T	13	P	X
15	C	M	S	F
A	17	K	B	M
X	A	L	19	E

</td><td>

12	C	B	K	F
S	V	14	A	R
T	16	R	X	B
F	W	T	18	E
20	A	B	Y	T

</td></tr>
</table>

Stand or sit about four to six feet back from the imaginary *X*. Move your eyes up to the letter *L* in the upper left-hand corner. Now slowly and systematically read to yourself the adjacent letters and number "1 U K T." Use your peripheral vision horizontally to the right in order to locate the letter *C* in the right-hand upper quadrant. Slowly and systematically read the adjacent letters and number "2 S O H." Now use your peripheral vision vertically downwards to locate the number 12 in the right-hand lower quadrant. Slowly and systematically read the adjacent letters "C B K F."

Now use your peripheral vision horizontally to the left to locate the letter *M* in the left-hand lower quadrant. Slowly and systematically read the adjacent letters and number "P O E 11." Now use your peripheral vision vertically upwards. But this time, don't start with the first letter *L*. Instead locate the letter *B* that is one line down in the left-hand upper quadrant. Slowly and systematically read the adjacent letters and number "P G 3 S." Repeat this pattern going around the four quadrants in a clockwise fashion. But each time you return to the upper left-hand quadrant, move down one line. Build from being able to do this, as tolerated, from thirty seconds to two minutes per session, two to three times per day (if evenings are hard on you, you can skip it).

If this brings on a lot of symptoms or it is very difficult to do, perform this exercise lying flat on your back, with the pattern stuck to the ceiling. If you are still too symptomatic or you can't do the exercise properly, perform the exercise with one eye covered by a towel, alternating eyes.

<u>Here is how to progress this exercise</u> (you don't need to do all variations given)**:**

1. If you have had to start doing this exercise one-eyed and lying on your back, progress to being able to do it with both eyes and on your back.

2. If you've had to start doing this exercise with both eyes and lying on your back, progress to sitting supported with a backrest, then to sitting unsupported, then, finally, to standing.

3. Now read the five-by-five letters counterclockwise and in reverse order (i.e., from right to left).

4. Now read faster. Don't read so fast that you can't keep the letters in focus, or you won't be accurate.

5. Now skip the numbers and only read the letters (80) as you move your way clockwise around the square.

6. Do variation number 5 but backwards (i.e., reading left to right and moving around the quadrants in a counterclockwise direction).

7. Now skip the letters and only read the numbers (20) as you move your way clockwise around the square. To do this, your eyes will need to move farther and more randomly.

8. Do variation number seven but backwards (i.e., reading left to right and moving around the quadrants in a counterclockwise direction).

9. Do exercise variations three through eight while doing balance exercises (see above). Do this by placing your feet in progressively harder positions (see positional pictures in the "Version—Smooth Pursuit" exercise above, page X). Make sure you have a chair back in front of you so you can hold it if you start to lose your balance. You do not want to jar yourself by falling!

10. Do exercise variations three through eight while using a metronome to set your pace. With each beat of the metronome, say the letter in your mind or out loud.

Start at a slow beat (i.e., fifty to sixty bpm) and gradually build as tolerated to a higher speed (i.e., 100-120 bpm). Make sure you have a chair back in front of you so you can hold it if you start to lose your balance. You do not want to jar yourself by falling!

11. Do exercise variations three through eight with your head turned fully, but comfortably, to the right, then to the left.

12. Do exercise variations three through eight with the five-by-five letter blocks stuck onto a demanding visual background (e.g., busy wallpaper).

13. Do exercise variations three through eight with an added noise distraction (e.g., while listening to some harmonious music or a conversation on the radio/TV).

<u>Day-to-Day Practices</u> (in order of difficulty)

Use your imagination. The following are just a couple of examples using this skill. Make sure to hold your head still and keep a good, elongated, standing/sitting posture (i.e., as if you are a puppet and someone has pulled your centre string).

For small-scale saccadic eye motions, read a large print book or e-book. Progress to smaller lettering, then to reading on a large regular screen, and finally to reading on a mobile phone.

- For small to medium saccadic eye motions, read the numbers of a traditional large-faced kitchen clock, clockwise and then counterclockwise.

- For medium to large saccadic eye motions, stand in front of a wall and move your eyes from one corner where the wall meets the ceiling to the other corner, then down to the floor's corner and back to the other floor's corner. Do this first clockwise, then counterclockwise.

You can make all of these day-to-day activities harder if you do them for progressively longer times, stand rather than sit, randomly change direction, safely challenge your balance (see above), and/or add noise or brighter light to the task.

2. Vergence – Convergence and Divergence Exercises

Do this exercise if Test 4 and/or Test 5 bring(s) on only a mild or mild-to-moderate increase in your symptoms. You should consult a neuro-optometrist if you experience any double vision with a target greater than twelve to fifteen centimeters from your nose.

Start by making yourself two targets. For the first target, draw a thick vertical line with a black marker on a plain stick (like a capital *I*, but without the top and bottom bars, "I"). Alternatively (but not quite as good), you can use your index finger as this first target. To make the second target, draw a similar but taller and thicker line in the middle of a sticky note (aka a Post-it note).

- If your balance is poor, or you're dizzy, do this exercise seated.
- At eye level on a wall, place a sticky note with a vertical line. Stand back about 245 centimeters (8 feet).
- At arm's length, hold a stick with a similar line on it. Focus on its line. Then shift your gaze to the sticky note's.
- Make sure the lines are single before moving on.
- Keeping shifting your eyes from one target to the other.

For a video of this, see
https://www.paulgodlewski.com/concussion-vision-issues

Try to keep your eyes properly focused on the sticky note's vertical line for a full count of five seconds (I like to count animals: one aardvark, two aardvarks …). Build from three sets of three repetitions (with a break between each set) to three sets of ten repetitions, two to three times per day (if evenings are hard on you, just do the exercises earlier twice a day).

If you are finding this visual task brings on a lot of symptoms or it is very difficult to do, try to relax your mind and body with some deep breathing, then blink your eyes. If it's still hard, move the popsicle stick and the sticky note a bit further away until you are able to do this. Up to twelve to fifteen centimeters is fine for the closer target. If you need to move it beyond twelve to fifteen centimeters, it's best you consult a neuro-optometrist.

<u>Here is how to progress this exercise</u>:
- If, in order to focus properly (without double vision) on the vertical line, you've had to move the stick farther than ten centimeters away from your nose, your first step is to gradually bring the stick back to the ten-centimeter distance from the nose.
- Assuming you have succeeded in holding the stick about ten centimeters from your nose while doing three sets of ten repetitions, two to three times per day, then progress by gradually moving the popsicle stick closer (up to six centimeters is good). As in all neuroplastic exercises, quality, not quantity, is more important.
- Now flick your eyes back and forth faster between the two targets. Don't go so fast that you are not able to properly focus on the vertical lines either close up or further away.

- Do the exercise while performing balance exercises (i.e., multitasking). Do this by placing your feet in progressively harder positions (see positional pictures in the "Version—Smooth Pursuit" exercise above). Make sure you have a chair back in front of you so you can hold onto it if you start to lose your balance. You don't want to jar yourself by falling!
- Do the exercise with your head turned fully, but comfortably, to the right, then to the left.
- Do the exercise with the sticky note stuck onto a demanding visual background (e.g., busy wallpaper).
- Do the exercise with an added noise distraction (e.g., while listening to some harmonious music or a conversation on the radio/TV).

<u>Day-to Day Practices</u> (in order of difficulty)

Use your imagination. The following are just a few ways to use these skills. Make sure to hold your head still and keep a good, elongated sitting posture (i.e., as if you are a puppet and someone has pulled your centre string) with your back supported.

1. At home, as tolerated, practice looking at a nearby object, then at one farther away, at varying distances (e.g., back and forth between your hands, resting on your lap, and then to a nearby lamp), and for increasing amounts of time. Make sure that the given target comes into focus and isn't doubled before returning to the other target.
2. Do the same as 1, but with your back unsupported (e.g., sitting on your bed).
3. Do the same as 2, but flicking your eyes forward and back more quickly, as tolerated.
4. Now do it out in the community with increasing distances, brighter light levels, and higher sound levels.

5. Do the exercise in a moving car (with someone else driving!). For example, take a page with a series of coloured squares. With the page on your lap, first look at one square—let's say the red square. Now look through the front windshield for roughly the same colour somewhere in front of your car. Make sure a given target comes into focus before returning to the page. Alternatively, instead of coloured squares, you can use numbers, shapes, or letters on the page, and try to find something like that ahead of you.

6. Do the same as 5 but, as tolerated, do it while looking out a side window of the travelling car.

Visual Perception Exercises

Visual perception is a complex process involving interacting parts. Together, your brain knits these skills together to give you visual perception. As you can imagine, testing and treating visual perception are beyond what you should be undertaking on your own. This can be very tricky as losses in any of these capacities can be quite subtle. So, you may not even be aware that you're struggling with this. Two things can help you know if visual perception may be an issue for you:

- If you're having real difficulty progressing the previous exercises, it may be the result of these subtle changes in your visual perceptual ability.

- The exercises that follow may also give some insight that you are struggling with visual perception. In either of these cases, it's worthwhile to consult a neuro-optometrist.

Exercise 1. Start by making a coloured photocopy from the website noted below of Appendix H "Letters, Numbers, Shapes, and Colours."

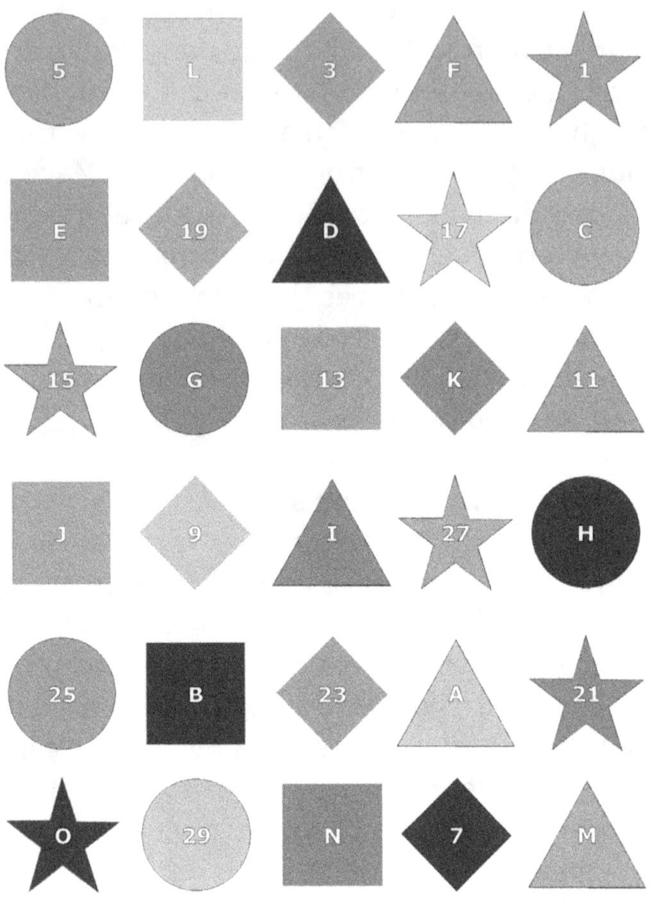

Appendix H in colour is only available at
https://www.paulgodlewski.com/concussion-exercise-tools-
and-appendices/

Tape the coloured sheet so that the centre of the sheet
is at eye level. Usually, this exercise is done while
standing. But if your balance is poor or this makes you
dizzy, start doing it while seated. Wearing your glasses,
if needed, stand or sit about 100 centimeters to 120

centimeters back from the sheet. Make sure to hold your head still and keep a good, elongated standing/sitting posture (i.e., as if you are a puppet and someone has pulled your centre string). If you find this brings on a lot of symptoms or is very difficult to do, try to relax your mind and body with some deep breathing, then blink your eyes.

- Scan the picture in order of the odd numbers (one, three, five, etcetera), saying each number to yourself.
- Scan the picture in order of the letters (A, B, C, etcetera), saying each letter to yourself.

As tolerated, build from being able to do this for thirty seconds to two minutes, two to three times per day (if evenings are hard on you, just do the exercises earlier twice per day). You can progress to a harder level once you can remember where the various numbers are located (more or less) and can tolerate doing this for two minutes.

<u>Here is how to progress this exercise</u>:
- Scan the picture in order of the odd numbers (one, three, five, etcetera), but instead of saying each number to yourself, say to yourself the shape the number sits in (i.e., star, diamond, circle, etcetera). Alternatively, say the colour of the shape the number sits in (i.e., purple, purple, red, etcetera). Scan the picture in order of the letters (A, B, C, etcetera), but instead of saying each letter to yourself, say to yourself the shape the letter sits in (i.e., triangle, square, circle, etcetera). Alternatively, say the colour of the shape the number sits in (i.e., yellow, brown, green, etcetera).
- Scan the picture in order, but alternate between finding and saying the odd numbers to yourself with

finding and saying the letters to yourself (i.e., one, A, three, B, five, C, etcetera).

- Scan the picture in order of the odd numbers, but instead of reading each number to yourself, alternate between saying the shape to yourself and saying the colour to yourself (i.e., star, purple, circle, brown, etcetera). Scan the picture in order of the letters, but instead of reading each letter to yourself, alternate between saying the shape to yourself and saying the colour to yourself (i.e., triangle, brown, circle, brown, etcetera).

- Scan the picture, alternating the order of the odd numbers and letters (i.e., one, A, three, B, five, C, etcetera). But instead of reading each odd number or letter to yourself, say the corresponding shape to yourself (i.e., star, triangle, diamond, square, circle, circle, etcetera). Scan the picture, alternating the order of the odd numbers and letters (i.e., one, A, three, B, five, C, etcetera). But instead of reading each odd number or letter to yourself, say the corresponding colour to yourself (i.e., purple, yellow, purple, brown, red, green, etcetera).

- Scan the picture, alternating the order of the odd numbers and letters (i.e., one, A, three, B, five, C, etcetera). But instead, alternate saying to yourself the odd number, then the shape of the first letter, then the next number, then the colour of the next letter (i.e., one, triangle, three, brown, five, circle, etcetera). Scan the picture, alternating the order of the letters and the odd numbers (i.e., A, one, B, three, C, five, etcetera). But instead, alternate saying to yourself the letter, then the colour of the first number, then the next letter, then the shape of the next number (i.e., A, purple, B, diamond, C, red, etcetera).

- Scan the picture, alternating the order of the odd numbers and letters but backwards (i.e., twenty-nine, O, twenty-seven, N, twenty-five, M, etcetera). Alternate saying to yourself the odd number, then the shape of the letter, then the next number, and then the colour of the next letter (i.e., twenty-nine, star, twenty-seven, blue, twenty-five, triangle, etcetera). You can make any of these levels more difficult by adding progressively more distracting background noise (e.g., listening to some quiet harmonious music versus louder conversation from a radio/TV).

Bear in mind these tasks, especially at the higher levels, would be challenging for anyone. Don't think you have to perfect this quickly. On the other hand, if, after many tries (persevere!), you simply can't advance through the levels, especially the lower ones, this may be a clue that you need further investigation by a neuro-optometrist.

Exercise 2. Jigsaw puzzles are a fun way to exercise many of the components of visual perception, including figure-ground delineation, visual discrimination, visual spatial relationships, visual closure, visual spatial memory, and visualization.

Purchase a jigsaw puzzle of approximately twenty to thirty largish pieces. The overall picture should be a simple clear drawing, with high contrast and bold colours. If possible, set the puzzle up on a table where you can leave it undisturbed, with good nonflickering lighting. Alternatively, place it on a large board so you can move it elsewhere as needed. Make sure to hold your head still and keep a good, elongated sitting posture (i.e., as if you are a puppet and someone has pulled your centre string) with your back supported. As tolerated, build from being able to do this for five to thirty minutes, once per day. You can progress to harder puzzles once you can do thirty minutes solidly once per day.

Here is how to progress this exercise:
- Use a puzzle with more pieces
- Do the puzzle with your back unsupported
- Increase the difficulty of the picture (i.e., lower contrast, more muted colours)
- Do the exercise with an added noise distraction (e.g., while listening to some harmonious music or a conversation on the radio/TV)

Day-to-Day Practices

No one activity can possibly work and improve all the components of visual perception. Fortunately, almost anything you do in your activities of daily living will exercise your visual perceptual skills.

7.8 When Not to Go It Alone

There are a number of instances following a concussion in which you should *not* contemplate doing vision exercises without expert advice. Remember, none of this information should be used in any way to self-diagnose. You should *not* try these exercises
- if your ophthalmologist or optometrist has found some structural eye or nerve issues (i.e., problems with your cornea, iris, lenses, retina optic nerve, eye pressure, and/or your visual field);
- if you are aware of any areas in your field of vision that you can't make out well;
- if you have difficulty discriminating objects from their background;

- if you have difficulty deciding what an object is or what it is used for;
- if you find yourself frequently bumping into things to the side of you and/or above you (this may be a sign of a midline shift in your sense of where you are in space);
- if you find it very hard to walk without side-stepping and/or losing your balance;
- If during Test 5 (convergence), you see double at greater than fifteen centimeters from your nose; and/or
- if any of the tests bring on a severe increase in your symptoms (i.e., 4 to 5/5).

If none of these applies to you, it's worthwhile to try the exercises. They may eventually help you reduce your symptoms with day-to-day visual tasks and do such tasks with greater ease and, gradually, for longer periods (e.g., tolerating reading longer), in addition to being able to accomplish increasingly harder visual tasks (e.g., reading on a computer). This will take time! If you see no improvement after six to eight weeks of doing the following exercises *regularly*, you should consult a neuro-optometrist.

Alternatively, if you're overwhelmed at the prospect of doing these exercises by yourself or if you know in your heart of hearts that you're not likely to persist on your own, you may want to consult a physiotherapist or occupational therapist who is *trained and experienced* in concussion rehabilitation, including basic vision therapy. You may also want to consult a therapist if you have done the exercises but you want to progress further toward your recovery.

With all rehabilitation exercises, it's very important that you not just repeat the same level of exercise over and over. As tolerated, challenge yourself gradually by doing them more often and at a harder level. In addition, try to work these skills into real, everyday activities too. If you don't practice these things in real life, you may just get good at doing the exercises. For most of the exercises, under the title "Day-to-Day Practices," I have included real-life examples where you can practice the skill. You apply these skills all the time in day-to-day activities, so use your imagination.

References

1. Ciuffreda, K. and Ludlam, D. 2011. "Conceptual Model of Optometric Vision Care in Mild Traumatic Brain Injury." *Journal of Behavioural Optometry*. 22, no 1 (Jan). https://www.researchgate.net/publication/268172783
2. Padula, W.V., et al. 2017. "The Consequence of Spatial Visual Processing Dysfunction Caused by Traumatic Brain Injury (TBI)." *Brain Inj.* 31 no 5 (Apr),589-600. https://doi.org/10.1080/02699052.2017.1291991
3. Hunt A. et al. 2016. "Oculomotor-Based Vision Assessment in Mild Traumatic Brain Injury: A Systematic Review." *Journal of Head Trauma Rehabilitation*. 31, no. 4 (Jul-Aug), 252-261. https://doi.org/10.1097/HTR.0000000000000174
4. Berger S. et al. 2016 "Effectiveness of Intervention to Address Visual and Visual-Perceptual Impairments to Improve Occupational Performance in Adults with Traumatic Brain Injury: A Systematic Review." *American Journal of Occupational Therapy.* 70 no 3 (May), 1-7. https://doi.org/10.5014/ajot.2016.020875
5. Simpson M. and Hunt A. 2019. "Vision Rehabilitation Interventions Following Mild Traumatic Brain Injury: A Scoping Review." *Disability and Rehabilitation.* 41 no. 18 (Sep): 2206-2222. https://doi.org/10.1080/09638288.2018.1460407

6. Thiagarajan P. et al. 2014. "Oculomotor Neurorehabilitation for Reading in Mild Traumatic Brain Injury (mTBI): An Integrative Approach." *NeuroRehabilitation.* 34 no 1, 129–146 https://doi.org/10.3233/NRE-131025

7. Thiagarajan P. and Ciuffreda K. 2013. "Effect of Oculomotor Rehabilitation on Vergence Responsivity in Mild Traumatic Brain Injury." *Journal of Rehabilitation Research and Development.* 50, no. 9,1223-40. https://doi.org/10.1682/JRRD.2012.12.0235

8. Thiagarajan P. and Ciuffreda K. 2014 "Effects of Oculomotor Rehabilitation on Accommodative Responsivity in Mild Traumatic Brain Injury." *Journal of Rehabilitation Research and Development.* 51, no 2, 175-191. https://doi.org/10.1682/JRRD.2013.01.0027

9. Thiagarajan P. and Ciuffreda K. 2014 "Versional Eye Tracking in Mild Traumatic Brain Injury (mTBI)." *Brain Injury.* 28, no. 7 (Mar) 930-943. https://doi.org/10.3109/02699052.2014.888761

10. Thiagarajan P. and Ciuffreda K. 2015. "Short-Term Persistence of Oculomotor Rehabilitative Changes in Mild Traumatic Brain Injury." *Brain Injury.* 29, no. 12 (Aug), 1475-1479. https://doi.org/10.3109/02699052.2015.1070905

Part 3

How to Get Back to What You
Want and Need to Do

Chapter 8

How to Get Back to School and/or Work

"The person who moves a mountain begins by carrying away small stones." Confucius

Cheat Sheet

8.1 How Alfred Managed to Return to His Work
During a volleyball game, Alfred was struck forcibly in the forehead by the ball. It took seven months of home exercises, work conditioning, and graduated return for him to resume his work as a nurse.

8.2 When to Not Go It Alone
When it comes to returning to activity, whether recreation, sport, studies, or work, it's best not to go it alone.

8.3 Ah, Mom, Do I Really Have to Go Back to School?!
Acquiring skills and knowledge is a child's primary form of work. However, getting them back to it as soon as possible should not be the goal. Instead, the goal should be a *successful* return to school.

8.4 General Recommendations for a Return to Learning

The 2022 Amsterdam Consensus Statement provides the foundational document for how we return concussed students to learning. This is regardless of the how the injury occurred.

8.5 Return to Primary School (i.e., ages five to twelve, grades one to seven)

When it comes to returning primary school children, CanChild has a wonderful set of tools to inform clinicians, teachers, and parents how best to get children back to school.

8.6 Return to Secondary School (i.e., ages thirteen to seventeen, grades eight to twelve)

The Living Guideline for Pediatric Concussion Care provides great guidance for returning older children and teens to school or work. I outline what you can find in this tool and provide the links to it.

8.7 When the Back-to-School Plan Is Not Going to Plan

This section outlines what to do if, despite everyone's best effort, your child is struggling to return to school.

8.8 Return to Post-Secondary Studies (i.e., age eighteen and up, college or university)

The Ontario Neurotrauma Foundation (ONF) has a separate parent/student version meant for students eighteen and over. I outline what you can find in this tool and provide the links to it.

8.9 So, You Wanna Get Back to Work. Well, Do Ya?

The first step in getting back to work is deciding what you want to get back to. Some take the opportunity to change their priorities and work/life mix. Others don't have this freedom and just need to get back.

8.10 What I Think Works Best for Getting Patients Back to Work

Based on my experience getting my own patients back to work in a large variety of settings, this section provides details on how to go about doing this. This is much more successful than rushing or winging it.

8.1 How Alfred Managed to Return to His Work

One weekend while playing beach volleyball, Alfred was struck in the forehead with a smash strike from the opposing team. He fell forward onto the sand and struck his forehead again on his elbow. He was dazed for some moments but did not lose consciousness. He was able to get up unassisted. The opposition team player who struck him drove him to emergency. All the tests came back normal, and he was instructed by the emergency doctor to rest, take time off work, and consult his GP.

As he knew they were very short-staffed at his hospital, he tried the next day to resume his work as a triage nurse in his hospital's emergency department. He was not able to cope, so he left work and consulted his GP. She diagnosed a concussion and referred him to a multidisciplinary

249

concussion program. On assessment, he reported in order of severity the following symptoms: head pressure but no headache, sleep disturbance, sensitivity to light, fogginess, dizziness, and difficulty remembering and concentrating.

The first twelve weeks of his recovery were spent doing home exercises and intermittently consulting clinicians. Although preferred by the PT, his employer was unable to allow him to do work shadowing as preparation for return to work. As an alternative, the PT suggested work-mimicking outside of his work for four weeks (see below). The graduated return process took an additional twelve weeks. His health care team strongly advised against returning sooner, as the prescribed time was typical for many in demanding work settings.

Later, he told his PT that he was very grateful for the time the team had insisted on, as he found the initial three to four weeks very hard going indeed. He resumed his shifting schedule only when the graduated return to his previous hours was complete. In the end, it was seven months before he was able to resume his full-time full duties, including shift work.

8.2 When Not to Go It Alone

In this chapter and the next, I'm breaking format and moving this section near to the top. The most important thing to understand is that you should not *go it alone when returning to activity*, whether for recreation, sport, studies, or work. As a minimum, you need the advice of a family doctor. But medical practitioners will vary in their detailed knowledge of what may be best practice for a concussion. It's better to consult a qualified health care practitioner (s) (e.g., sport MD, PT, OT, etcetera) knowledgeable about evidence-based concussion management.

A knowledgeable patient or patient's advocate is also a key member of the team. To that end, in this chapter I will provide you with the tools to be a knowledgeable health care consumer. This is not to encourage you to manage alone your return to learning, return to work, etc., but to help you better understand the process and to know what questions to ask your qualified health care practitioner (s) or qHCP.

In the first section, I will go over some general recommendations about returning to activity. Thereafter, I start with children going back to primary school after a concussion, then post-secondary students, and finish with adults returning to work. The return-to-school sections are, for the most part, directing you to some excellent resources. As there is less material available, the last section on adults returning to work relies more heavily on my own experience of what works best.

8.3 Ah, Mom, Do I Really Have to Go Back to School?!

No doubt, this is a very common question from children, whether or not they have a concussion. For the most part, the answer is most emphatically yes! Acquiring skills and knowledge is of primary importance to children. But getting them back to it as soon as possible shouldn't be the goal. Instead, the goal should be a *successful* return to school. Success is measured by both their ability to tolerate the return and, importantly, their capacity to absorb and learn.

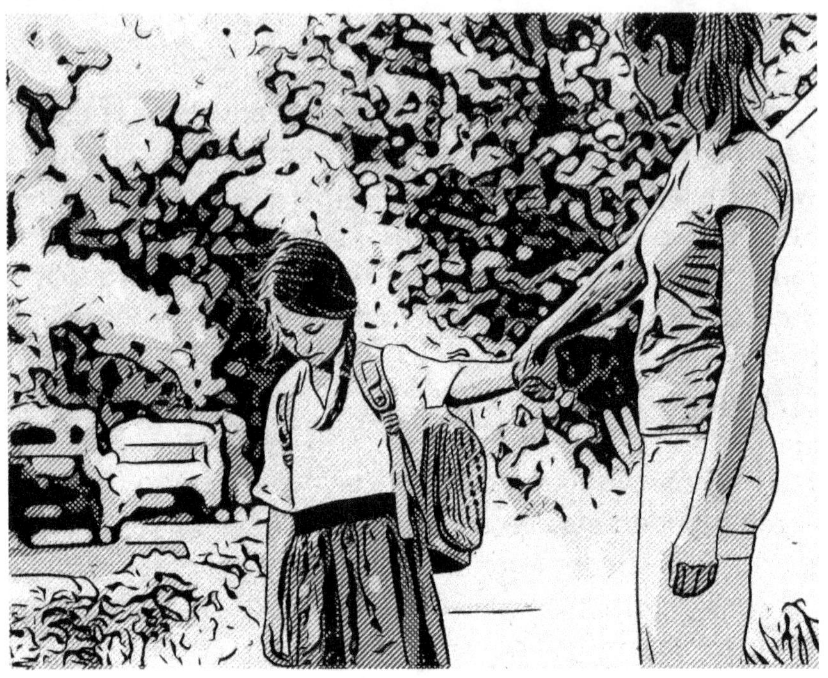

I will start by giving you some up-to-date general recommendations (see section 8.4) for returning to learning. Beyond this, there are some wonderful age-specific resources out there. Rather than try to reinvent the wheel, I am going to point you to those I've found are the most useful for my patients. Based on the student's age, these resources flesh out things in a way the general recommendation cannot. The URLs for these resources have a habit of changing. This makes it hard sometimes for readers to find the resources. To this end, in the references, I provide you with the date when I last accessed the site, as well as the name of the resource.

8.4 General Recommendations for a Return to Learning

These general recommendations are based on the 2023 Amsterdam Consensus Statement on Concussion in Sport.[1] However, they can still be used for concussion coming from other types of injuries (e.g., a fall).

- In order to facilitate a successful return to leaning, all those involved with the student (i.e., parents, educators, and clinicians) need to work together.
- Not all students will need tailored academic supports or a return-to-learning (RTL) strategy.
- If return to learning is more prolonged than expected, then academic supports need to be put into place to overcome barriers. These include changing the environment, the physical activity, and the curricular and testing factors.
- An RTL strategy should be considered if
  - the student's symptoms continue to be worsened by cognitive activity and screen time; and/or
  - the student has difficulty with reading, concentration, memory, and other aspects of learning.

For those students needing a RTL strategy, the consensus document recommends the following steps: [2]

<u>Step 1</u>
It's often best to start with a period of twenty-four to forty-eight hours of relative rest.

For all the next steps, there should be only a mild increase in symptoms (i.e., a two on a scale of ten, where zero is no symptoms and ten is the worst symptoms imaginable). In addition, this increase should last for less than one hour. If this is not achieved, the progress within, and between, the steps need to be slowed down.

Step 2
The concussed student resumes their typical non-study activities. Start them with five to fifteen minutes of a given activity and increase gradually.

Step 3
The concussed student gradually brings on activities that prepare them to return to formal studies. For example: homework, reading, etcetera.

Step 4
The concussed student returns to formal studies part-time (i.e., a limited number of study periods or a greater number of rest periods). Gradually, they should increase the number of study periods and/or decrease their rest periods.

Step 5
The concussed student returns to formal studies full-time, including catching up on missed material.

The general recommendations contained in this section are a very good foundation for how to return a child, or youth, to learning. But such provisions can be tricky to apply to different ages and situations. To this end, the following sections provide age-specific resources. If there is a contradiction between one guideline and another, I suggest you use the most up-to-date guideline. As we learn more, naturally, our knowledge and practices need to evolve.

8.5 Return to Primary School (i.e., ages five to twelve, grades one to seven)

How quickly a child recovers depends on many factors, including the severity of their concussion, whether they experienced concussion-associated amnesia, the number of concussions they have had, the symptoms of ongoing fogginess and/or dizziness, the presence of migraines before or after the concussion, and a prior history of learning or behavioural problems. Using one-size-fits-all templates for all children *does not* work.

However, parents often needlessly worry when their child continues to report symptoms while returning to school. Children do not need to be symptom-free to begin the return to school process and to progress well. Nevertheless, it is very important that all parties involved (parents, educators, and clinicians) regularly check in with the child to find out how they are feeling and coping. Everyone, especially the child, needs to know that ignoring symptoms (i.e., the "suck it up" approach) is not a good idea. It can lead to prolonged issues and, in some cases, completely stall recovery.

The MacMaster's CanChild guide for concussed children[3] has a robust and straightforward return-to- school guide for clinicians, teachers, and parents to help get children back to school. It outlines five distinct stages and includes when to move forward to the next stage or to move back to the previous level. CanChild recommends a full return to school before starting three additional stages to return to sport.

I'm frequently asked by the parents of my younger patients, "How long is it going to take for my child to feel better?" The pat answer is "It depends" (see the above factors). But a better way to answer this is with these helpful statistics from an earlier version of McMaster University's *CanChild's Return to School Guidelines.* On average, the time it takes is fifteen days for 25 percent, twenty-six days for 50 percent, forty-five days for 75 percent, and ninety-two days for 90 percent of concussed children to be symptom-free. Bear in mind that statistics are forever being refined and updated. Still, this will give you a general sense of the timelines involved, and be reassuring for parents. At the same time, they need to understand that, in some cases, it can take longer.

8.6 Return to Secondary School (i.e., ages thirteen to seventeen, grades eight to twelve)

The Living Guideline for Pediatric Concussion Care[4] also has a series of guides for children and teens returning to school. There is overlap with it and the CanChild guideline for the lower ages. For the lower ages, I prefer the CanChild guide, as the parents and children of my practice have found it easier to use.

8.7 When the Back-to-School Plan Is Not Going to Plan

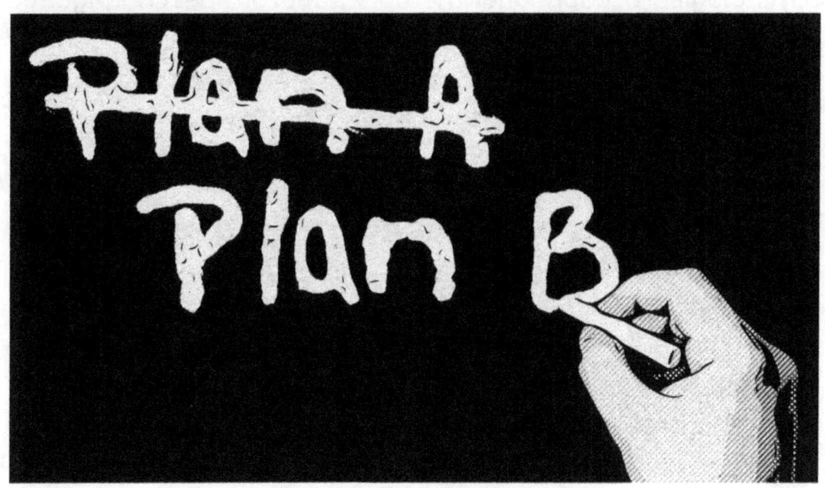

So, it has been a while since the concussion, and things don't seem to be getting that much better for your child or, if anything, they seem to be worsening (i.e., increasing symptoms, decreasing concentration and/or increasing behavioural problems).

This is one of those times when professional help is especially important. Beyond the child's pediatrician, seek out professional help within the school system, or failing that, seek help outside it. There may be unidentified barriers to your child's progress that the concussion is now revealing or highlighting. These can include depression, anxiety, and/or learning disorders (e.g., attention deficit hyperactivity disorder – ADHD).

It's important to understand that a student can be diagnosed with the term ADHD even if they don't have all the components of the disorder. For example, if they're not particularly prone to hyperactivity, the child's school accommodations may need to be significantly increased, with the assistance of professionals (i.e., pediatric psychologist, occupational therapist, and/or speech language pathologist). These accommodations shouldn't be generic but must be carefully tailored to the child, with active participation from their parents and teachers.

8.8 Return to Post-Secondary Studies (i.e., age eighteen and up, college or university)

Older students need a different approach to returning to studies after concussion. This is not only because they have the greater agency of adults, but also because their brains are different from those of a child or younger teen. To this end, the *Concussion Ontario* has a separate series of documents meant for those eighteen and over.[5]

The mental and physical exertion needs to be managed carefully to avoid going above tolerance and/or prolonging symptoms. But because you're dealing with adults, it can be handled in a more nuanced way (see chapters 3 and 4). To aid the return to college or university, the student or their caregiver must notify their school registrar as soon as possible. Thereafter, they need to work closely with all their instructors and, if the concussion/PPCS is more prolonged and/or severe, the institution's disabilities and health services.

8.9 So, You Wanna Get Back to Work. Well, Do Ya?

I am not being entirely flippant with this question. For many of my patients, the enforced slowdown necessitated by their concussion or PPCS gives them the opportunity to revaluate what they are doing. Do they really want to be as busy and stressed as before? Some take the opportunity to change their priorities and rebalance their work/life mix. For others, they just want to, or have to, get back to what they were doing before. For sure, getting back to work is the priority for most people. They want to resume their roles and responsibilities and earn income. But this is not all. Getting back to work turns out to be better for you as well as your brain.[6]

Let's assume you're trying to get back to your pre-concussion work. I will start with some general recommendations. After that, I'll flesh these out with what I have found works best, along with some examples to make it clearer. *Concussion Ontario* has a patient version for return to work, section 12 (b) *"Return-to-Activity - Work Consideration."* [6]

While it's true some individuals would really prefer not to return to work, in my experience, the vast majority of individuals genuinely want to return. If anything, as a clinician, I more often act as a brake: getting them to prepare better for their return, slow down how fast they come back, and/or modify the duties they reassume. The biggest factors leading to failure in returning to work are:
- inadequate prior preparation before starting the return-to-work process;
- an overall poorly managed process either from inside and/or outside the work;
- too quickly ramping up hours and duties; and/or
- inadequate early-on accommodations.

The clinician's version of the *Concussion Ontario* return to work document lists the following common accommodations to help workers return successfully: [6]

- Assistance with commuting to and from work
- Flexible work hours (e.g., starting later or ending earlier)
- Gradual work re-entry (e.g., starting at two half days per week and expanding gradually).
- Additional time for task completion
- Having a quiet space available for breaks throughout the day
- A temporary change of duties
- Environmental modifications
  o quieter work environment
  o enhanced level of supervision
  o decreased computer work
  o ability to work from home
  o only day-shift hours

These are all very good recommendations. But again, like return to learning, getting back to work with a concussion or PPCS can be quite tricky. In the next section, I will discuss what I have found increases the chance of a successful return to work. Bear in mind this is just my experience, and level four on scale of evidence outline in the Introduction.

8.10 What I Have Found Works Best for Getting Patients Back to Work

When a worker has injured their back or shoulder, it's common to prepare them with work conditioning and, in some cases, work hardening. For concussions, and particularly PPCS, preparation for return to work is often overlooked. It should be no different with a brain injury. It's best to think of this preparation as a functional extension of the exercises mapped out in the earlier chapters. The concussion patient must be able to transform the isolated skills in these exercises into the multidimensional combination of skills needed for work. It's even more important to prepare the individual for doing these tasks in a variety of different environments, especially often challenging or nonoptimal environments (e.g., busy and noisy).

When possible, it's best to use a two-step approach to returning patients to work.
- Work conditioning to prepare the person for a return to work.
- Begin a graduated return to work through modification of duties and accommodations.

While not all concussed workers will need a work-conditioning phase, most in my experience benefit from this. Inadequate or rushed preparation for the working environment is why so many return plans fail. Disability managers and employers frequently underestimate the importance of this work-conditioning phase and the time it will take.

Work Conditioning
<u>Work Mimicking</u>
In broad strokes, the key to this process is understanding what the individual will face on their return to work— what kind of tasks, environments, and commuting or travelling it will involve. In a nutshell, work mimicking involves getting the individual to build tolerance and capacity for:
- doing work-like tasks, matched as much as possible to what they do;
- spending more and more time doing these work-like activities;

- working in progressively more challenging environments; and
- commuting progressively farther away from home to match their actual commute.

Sometimes, work mimicking is relatively easy to reproduce. In other cases, due to the nature of the person's job, the work may be virtually impossible to duplicate.

An example will make all this much clearer. Let's return to the case of emergency triage nurse Alfred outlined at the beginning of this chapter. Alfred's job requires him to cope with multiple stressors. Physically, he needs to be able to sit for long periods of time viewing a computer screen. Cognitively, he has to do a lot of triage-thinking (priority assessing and sorting of patients for care). Psychologically, he needs to interact frequently with very stressed, unhappy and demanding patients. Environmentally, he needs to be able to work with his fellow doctors and nurses in an often-busy, noisy, fluorescent-lit environment.

His pre-concussion schedule was eight hours a day, five days per week, rotating every two weeks from daytime to evening to a graveyard shift. Before the concussion, he commuted to work via public transit fifty minutes each way. His job required that 75 percent of his time be in front of a computer screen (interviewing patients), 15 percent of the time in one-to-one meetings consulting other health professionals (often on the move in corridors), and 10 percent of the time in larger staff meetings.

In his case, his work was easy to mimic for some things and almost impossible to reproduce for other aspects of his job. Optimally then, work shadowing would have worked best for him (see below). However, his employer was not able to accommodate work shadowing due to privacy and liability concerns. Therefore, the next best thing was to prepare him, as much as possible, via work mimicking.

At the outset, a goal was established to build his tolerance from one hour per day to four to five hours per day on Monday, Wednesday, and Friday before initiating a graduated return to work process (see further below). He started working at home on his own laptop (equipped with a free app called Flux, set to a pink background colour that he discovered was most restful) responding to personal emails and surfing the web. He initially worked for thirty minutes a day, then built to sixty minutes a day (with a five-minute break after twenty-five to thirty minutes). Thereafter, Monday, Wednesday, and Friday (see below), he commuted via public transit to public libraries that were increasingly distant from his home. Eventually, he built to commuting fifty minutes each way to a large central public library. On his non-work-mimicking days, he rested and continued to do his physiotherapy exercises.

Task/Projects
From a variety of options, which he worked out with his PT, he chose to focus on rotating between three tasks:
- Studying to pass the written portion of an exam to become a surgical nurse.
- Researching materials and contacting contractors (in writing and on the phone) about a kitchen project he and his wife had long contemplated. This also included working with a reference librarian to access design magazines, find appliance reviews, and research the pros and cons of different materials.
- Watching TED talks, then writing up summaries and checking himself later to see what he retained.

While working at the library, he also tried, as much as he was able, to mix up tasks to roughly target the percentage of the different activities he did while at work (e.g., he spent approximately 75 percent of his time working on on-screen). The only thing that could not be mimicked was the high and frequent stress to which he was exposed while dealing with emergency patients.

Environment
The last library he worked at was structured around a large, open atrium. It had a variety of environments. Similar to his work, it was lit predominantly by overhead fluorescent lighting. The top floors of the library were morgue-like in their quietness, while the ground floor was often noisy (including an occasional Salsa class—boy, have libraries changed!). There was also a café on the ground floor that during lunch periods provided an even nosier environment in which to try to work. He moved between these different environments, backing off to quieter regions when he became too symptomatic or tired. Overall, he gradually increased his time working and did the work in increasingly challenging environments.

Work Shadowing
If available, work shadowing is a wonderful way of preparing to return to work. As the name implies, the person shadows the individual(s) doing the work in their absence as a kind of knowledgeable assistant. As with work mimicking, they gradually increase their hours until they can manage four to five hours Monday, Wednesday, and Friday (see the explanation of this as a reservoir technique below), whereupon the graduated return to work can be initiated for the person's job.

The wonderful thing about work shadowing is that their time is limited to a schedule and to their tolerance. Not having ultimate responsibility means that the stress the concussed person is exposed to is much more manageable. In addition, if needed, they can miss a day or days if the task/environment is proving too challenging. Their tasks are the same tasks they will be doing on return to work, and the environment is what they will have to deal with on their return.

Unfortunately, there are many reasons, logistical and political, that sometimes make it infeasible to use work shadowing as a preliminary to a graduated return to work. However, when available, work shadowing is superior to work mimicking. The length of time needed for work mimicking or shadowing is highly variable. It depends on the severity of the concussion, the complexity of the job, and the nature and safety of the environment to which the individual needs to return.

For example, returning to a clerical job in a quiet office after a mild concussion is radically different from the challenge of returning to work as a police officer recovering from a severe concussion caused by an assault, along with its associated PTSD. This is one of the reasons why cookie-cutter approaches and standards for return-to-work periods, favoured by some institutions, *do not work.*

Graduated Return to Work

As outlined previously (see chapter 3), concussions are understood as an energy crisis in the brain. For reasons not understood, the energy crisis very often continues into the PPCS phase. Pacing and planning are therefore key throughout the recovery period, not only for return to normal activities of daily living (ADLs) such as self-care, cooking, and cleaning, but also for what are called in the trade "instrumental activities of daily living" (IADLs) such as shopping, banking, studying, and working.

One very helpful technique for getting patients back to their more demanding IADLs (e.g., work) is combining a graduated return process along with built-in short and longer rest breaks, or what I call "energy rebuild reservoirs." The reservoir is a strategically placed mini and macro rest stop between times of greater activity. As the person recovers from their concussion/PPCS, the number and duration of these rest stops can be gradually diminished. The prearranged rest reservoirs allow the patient to gradually increase their tolerance to longer and longer periods of activity in a given day, and over the weeks.

After completing some activity conditioning (see above), the following schedule of breaks can be worked in as they build their time:

<u>Micro Breaks</u>
- For every twenty-five minutes of on-screen work, patients are instructed to take a five-minute break (e.g., a mini meditation, as detailed in chapter 3, or looking to the distance through a north window).
- For every cumulative two hours of work, they are instructed to take a fifteen-minute total break in an oasis spot (e.g., a sick room or unoccupied conference room).
- For every cumulative four hours of work, they are instructed to take an hour lunch break, preferably completely away from others and the work environment.

<u>Macro Breaks</u>

- Employers optimally should allow their returning concussion/PPCS employees to begin with just four hours per day, three days per week (Monday, Wednesday, Friday). This gives them two reservoir days during the week and two days on the weekend to recover. The first week(s) back are often the hardest for a concussed individual returning to work. For this reason, it's best if they remain at these hours for the first two weeks. Thereafter, keeping the reservoir days in place, they increase their work as tolerated hours, typically by one hour per day per week until they are working full-time on those workdays (i.e., Monday, Wednesday, Friday).

- Based on how they are doing, usually by the six- to seventh-week mark they can add four hours of work to both Tuesdays and Thursdays. Thereafter, they should increase by one hour per week until they are back full-time, Monday through Friday.

By far, the most difficult thing for an employer whose employee is off with a concussion/PPCS is the uncertainty of knowing when the employee will be returning, and how long it will take for them to be back up and running fully. As a clinician working in this area, unless the patient has a light concussion and will likely recover quickly, it's better to give monthly, rather than weekly, updates. This allows the employer to plan better and more realistically. Once the employee is ready to start the return, it's best, if possible, to give the employer an entire timeline for return to work.

As it's not always easy to estimate how this will go, it is important to book a midway reassessment to either slow, speed up, or hold the line on their return. Again, this makes it easier for employers to plan. Often, employers are not aware of and don't like the lengthy return process for brain injuries like concussions. But what employers dislike even more is employees coming and going due to flare-ups and improper and unrealistic planning.

Modification of Duties and Accommodations

A series of temporary modifications to the work environment can really aid a successful return to work.

These have to be tailored to the type of work. Some are easier to do in some work environments than others. Following are some of the most common modifications.

Screen Modifications

Modern-day work is dominated by large amounts of time in front of screens. Long periods of exposure to relatively high amplitude, high glare, blue-light-dominant spectrum and high frequency flickering are very challenging for most concussion and PPCS returning workers. There are at least seven workarounds from simple and inexpensive to more complex and costly. Ordered from cheaper to more expensive, they are as follows:

- Print out most material.
- Turn down the screen's brightness to the minimum or use sunglasses.
- Push back the monitor so it is occupying less of the field of vision.
- Install a colour-adapting app like Colorveil. Certain colours are more tolerated than others. These often-free apps allow the individual to experiment with what works best for them.
- Install an anti-glare screen in front of their monitor.

- Replace the monitor with a "low-flicker" screen version. There are a number available now.
- Replace the monitor with a "no flicker type." This takes the form of a usually somewhat smaller sized e-ink screen (e.g., Iris Monitor by Noviscend). These are excellent for reducing irritation from reading screens. Unfortunately, they are not always easy to source, are expensive, and don't handle video content well. Initially, it's a good idea to use them alongside a regular monitor. The former can be used for spreadsheets and other written documents, the latter for video and internet work.

Overhead Flickering Lighting and Floor Vibration
- It is not entirely clear why, but both consciously and unconsciously perceived flickering lights and vibrating floors pose a problem for concussed individuals. Likely it's related to vestibular gaze instability issues (see chapter 6), which pose significant challenges to most patients returning to work. For this reason, where possible, returning-to-work patients should limit their exposure to overhead fluorescent and certain types of LED lighting. This is easily achieved in a private office, where they can switch the lights off or replace them, if needed, with non-flickering LED or incandescent task lighting. In an open office, this is more challenging. In these cases, perhaps the employer can unscrew the fluorescent bulbs directly overhead. When not feasible, and if this is a big barrier to their capacity to cope and be productive, the employee may need to temporarily wear sunglasses and/or a baseball cap with a wide brim.
- Have the employee temporarily move into a private office or occupy a small meeting room.
- Some offices have raised floors that vibrate due to underlying A/C units. Similarly, some factories have a

lot of floor vibration associated with the running of heavy equipment. Theses situations need to be handled on a case-by-case basis.

Sound Sensitivity
Some patients may be more sound-sensitive than light-sensitive. When first getting back to work, they may need to work in more isolated areas. For example, a private office rather than an open office location.

Alternatively, they may need to employ sound-reducing earplugs strategically, as when the environment becomes very noisy or at the end of the work period when they are getting tired (see chapter 4).

Meetings
We take for granted so much of what our brains routinely do for us. One of these brain capacities is being able to cope with groups of people interacting and communicating. I like to use an example with my patients of the opera (which my wife so much enjoys, me, not so much). To be able to listen to the tenor or soprano soloist, you need to screen out or diminish your focus on the other singers. This is called sound zooming (see chapter 4). The need to do sound zooming is not confined to rarified locations like opera houses. It happens every time you're in a meeting. The more people you are actively interacting with in a meeting and the louder and more additional stimuli, the more screening and zooming you will need to do. Added to this is all the thinking and focus required in the meetings. Teleconferences incorporate a whole other dimension. You can see why meetings suck the gas out of those concussion/PPCS patients trying to return to work.

For this reason, patients should initially limit their interaction to one-on-one and small groups (i.e., two to three individuals). Thereafter, as tolerated, they can gradually interact with larger and larger groups. It's also helpful for patients to let the meeting chair and participants know in advance that they may need to limit the length of time in the meeting, or that they may need to step out from time to time. To that end, preferably and if possible, those items in the agenda that need the concussed person's direct input should be handled earlier in the session.

Avoidance of Shift Work and Overseas Work Trips
Both concussion and PPCS patients can have trouble with their sleep. The reasons for this are complex and multifactorial (see chapter 4). As a result, work requiring the patient to regularly alter their waking and sleeping cycle (i.e., shift work) should be avoided when initially returning to work. The same is true of work trips abroad, where the person is exposed to significant jet lag. How long these need to be avoided depends on a lot of factors, not least of which is ongoing concussion or other causes of sleep disturbance. As a rule of thumb, this accommodation should remain in place for at least the first eight to twelve weeks.

References

1. Patricios J.S., et al. 2023. "Consensus Statement on Concussion in Sport: The 6th International Conference on Concussion in Sport–Amsterdam. October 2022." Br J Sports Med. 57, no. 11 (Jun), 695–711. https://doi.org/10.1136/bjsports-2023-106898
2. Putukian, M. et al. 2023 "Clinical Recovery from Concussion: Return to School and Sport: A Systematic

Review and Meta-Analysis." *Br J Sports Med*. 57 no. 12 (Jun), 798-809. https://pubmed.ncbi.nlm.nih.gov/37316183/
3. CanChild. 2024. "Brain Injury Resources." https://www.canchild.ca/en/diagnoses/brain-injury-concussion/brain-injury-resources/
4. Pedsconcussion. 2024. "Pediatric Concussion Resources for Families, Schools, and Sports Organizations." https://www.pedsconcussion.com/tools-resources/community-resources/
5. Concussion Ontario. 2024. *Living Concussion Guidelines. Guideline for Concussion/Mild Traumatic Brain Injury and Prolonged Symptoms for Adults 18 years of age and older.* Patient version, section 12 a) *"Return-to-Activity – School.* Ontario Ministry of Health. Ministry of Long-Term Care. https://concussionsontario.org/concussion/patient-version/
6. Concussion Ontario. 2024. *Living Concussion Guidelines. Guideline for Concussion/Mild Traumatic Brain Injury and Prolonged Symptoms for Adults 18 years of age and older.* Patient version, section 12 b) *"Return-to-Activity – Work Considerations.* Ontario Ministry of Health. Ministry of Long-Term Care. https://concussionsontario.org/concussion/patient-version/

Chapter 9

How to Get Back to Sport and Recreation

"We hope all danger may be overcome. But to conclude that no danger may arise would itself be extremely dangerous." Abraham Lincoln

Cheat Sheet

9.1 How Dean Managed to Return to School and Hockey

During a hockey game, Dean was concussed by a much larger player checking him. His coach returned him to the game far too soon.

9.2 When Not to Go It Alone

While the contents of this chapter provide clear information about how best to return to recreation and sport, when it comes to returning to activity, you really should not try to go it alone.

9.3 Ah, Mom, When Do I Get to Play Again?!

Acquiring skills and knowledge is a child's primary form of work. However, getting them back to sport and active recreational activity is also very important for their development and well-being.

9.4 General Recommendations for a Return to Sport and Active Recreation

The 2022 Amsterdam Consensus Statement provides the foundational document for how we return to sport. This is regardless of the how the injury occurred. They can also be used for return to active recreational activities.

9.5 Returning Children to Activity

A one-size-fits-all template for all children *does not* work. McMaster's CanChild outlines six distinct stages of how and when to get children back to recreation and sport.

9.6 Returning Youth and Adults to Sport

Like the CanChild Guide above, Parachute's Return to Sport Strategy lays out six stages to return to sport for youth and adults. In addition, it provides a series of "sport-specific return-to-sport" guides.

9.7 Baseline Testing

Baseline tests are carried out for students before they start a given season of sport (usually team sports). With some noted exceptions, Parachute, a national charity dedicated to injury prevention, believes such testing is not useful.

9.1 How Dean Managed to Return to School and Hockey

Dean adores all things hockey, from watching hockey, to playing street shinny, to being on the ice. He has a somewhat more distant love in his life—summer baseball.

He is much less keen on high school. Nevertheless, prior to his injury he was doing okay academically. Despite being smallish for his age, he is usually able to hold his own playing at North America's "AAA midget level."

Early in the first period of a league game, he was checked into the boards by a much larger player, strongly jarring him. Dazed, he retreated to the bench and sat out the next period. The coach didn't witness the hit. Dean told him he was feeling much better. The coach wasn't sure he should let him back in the game but erroneously cleared him to resume play. Fortunately, the final period ended up being completely uneventful. A further incident could well have converted his then below-symptom-threshold injury into some thing far more serious.

As it happened, most of his symptoms came on the next morning: headaches, fatigue, fogginess, difficulty concentrating, sensitivity to sound, and a minor sensitivity to light. Unfortunately, this delay in symptom onset frequently happens in many concussions. Following a *possible* concussion event, his coach should have adhered to this rule:

A player should not return to play the same day!

and,

If in doubt, sit them out!

This time the coach, or more accurately the player, was lucky. Dean subsequently consulted his family doctor, who diagnosed a concussion and didn't consider any further imaging or other diagnostic tests necessary. Initially, he was just instructed to rest and sit the games out. The previous year, his doctor had diagnosed Dean with two concussions, each lasting two to three weeks. Before these incidents, Dean had had several brief concussion-like events, but they went undiagnosed, and each cleared in a few days.

This time, his doctor's first attempt to return Dean to school didn't work out due to symptoms and Dean's inability to cope with both the in-school work and home assignments. To help get him back to school and sport, his doctor referred him to a physiotherapist (PT) and an occupational therapist (OT) experienced in concussion management.

His physiotherapy treatments consisted of a specialized concussion cardio program (see chapter 3) to restore his cardio dysfunction and lessen his fatigue. In addition, he was given a mini meditation to calm his symptoms (see chapter 3), sleep hygiene education, instructed on how to use special earplugs in a time-limited fashion (see chapter 4), and static and dynamic balance exercises (see chapter 6). Finally, he was given some sport-specific drills to help him regain his capacity and test his readiness for a return to sport. The OT worked with him in pacing and planning (see chapter 3) and gave him a few progressive cognitive exercises to help him overcome the limited cognitive deficits she'd found in her assessment.

Working together, the PT and OT coordinated a gradual return, first to school, then to sport (see below). Overall, it took Dean six weeks to recover sufficiently to return fully to school. In collaboration with the information from his other clinicians, he was cleared by his sport doctor after three months to return to hockey, but only to practice. Given the timing of his concussion, the number of concussions or concussion-like events, and their increasing severity and recovery duration, he was advised by his sport MD against returning to competition until the next season.

That year, his team went on to the playoffs but lost, Dean claimed (only somewhat tongue in cheek), because of his absence in the lineup. The good news was that the added rest allowed him to return to hockey the next season without restrictions.

9.2 When to Not Go It Alone

This section and the next are very similar in content to the previous chapter. Again, I am breaking with format and moving this section up to the top. That's because the most important thing to understand is that *you should not to go it alone* when it comes to any return to sport and active recreational activities.

At a minimum, you need the advice and support of your family doctor. But medical practitioners will vary in their detailed knowledge of concussion best practice. Better to consult a qualified health care practitioner(s) or qHCP (e.g., sport MD, GP, PT, OT, etcetera) who is/are knowledgeable about evidence-based concussion management, as well as risk assessment. However, a knowledgeable patient or patient's advocate is key to a decision-making team. To that end, in this chapter I will provide you with the tools to be a knowledgeable health care consumer. This is not to encourage you to manage the return to activity alone, but to help you better understand the process and know what questions to ask your qualified health care practitioner (qHCP).

Risk assessment is a vitally important issue to consider in returning patients to sport. There is no one-size-fits-all to risk assessment. There are many factors that go into this assessment, including:

- The number of previous diagnosed concussions and concussion-like events.
- How severe the patient's concussions were and, assuming they recovered fully, how long it took.
- The degree of control the individual has over events in their sport. Team sports are generally considered much riskier for return than many individual sports, and some sports are much riskier than others.
- The gender of the individual and their age (e.g., teenage females are at greater risk of long-term injury and consequences than males of the same age).
- An inability to get back to school or work.
- Other physical and mental illnesses (aka comorbidities)—for example, physical disabilities or cognitive and psychiatric disorders.

Due to the very complex nature of these factors, I prefer to be part of a team of professionals collaborating to advise the patient and their families. When it comes to clearance to return to contact practice, it's especially important that this be done by an experienced physician, or a less experienced physician in consultation with other experienced rehab clinicians.

In the first sections, I will go over some general recommendations for return to sport and active recreation. These were initially designed specifically for sport but work well for return to many other forms of activity (e.g., return to recreation). I start with getting children back to activity (including sport), then move on to youth and adults trying to return to sport and active recreation. As a general rule, regardless of age, vigorous exertion or return to contact sport should be avoided while the concussed individuals are still recovering. Rather than try to reinvent the wheel, I am going to point to those resources I have found the most useful for my patients. Unfortunately, the URLs for these resources have a habit of changing, making them hard to find. To this end, I will provide you with the date when I last accessed the site, as well as the name of the resource.

9.3 Ah, Mom, When do I Get to Play Again?!

The consensus is that, for children and teens, the first priority is to successfully get them back to school. But some of the earlier stages of return to activity can happen at the same time as they are beginning to return to school. The later stages, however, should wait until they are fully back to school. Returning to sport and activity is important for physical and mental well-being as well as proper childhood development (oh, and also so they can blow off some steam and stop driving their parents crazy!).

9.4 General Recommendations for Return to Sport and Active Recreation

These general recommendations are based on the 2023 Amsterdam Consensus Statement on Concussion in Sport.[1] However, they can still be used for concussion coming from other types of injuries (e.g., a fall), as well as returning to other forms of physical recreation.

- All return to sport and recreation (RTSR) should be done under the supervision of a qualified health care practitioner (qHCP, see section 9.2).

- In order to facilitate a successful return to sport, all those involved with the student (i.e., parents, clinicians, and coaches) need to work together.
- Under the supervision of a qHCP, RTSR can be done in conjunction with return-to-learning steps (see chapter 8).
- *Players should not return to play on the same day* an incident occurs, because symptoms can take a while to develop. Thus, *"If in doubt, sit them out."* This applies to all concussed individuals, not just children and youth. Remember, one does not have to be struck on the head, lose consciousness, or have memory loss to have sustained a concussion.

Apart from step 1, there needs to be a minimum of twenty-four hours between each of the following steps:

Step 1
Start with a period of twenty-four to forty-eight hours of relative rest.

For RTSR steps 2-4, there should be only a mild increase in symptoms (i.e., two on a scale of ten, where zero is no symptoms and ten is the worst symptoms imaginable). In addition, this increase should last for less than one hour. If more than mild exacerbation of symptoms occurs during RTSR steps 2–4, the person should stop and attempt to exercise the next day. A concussed person experiencing concussion-related symptoms during RTSR steps 5–7 should return to step 4 to establish full resolution of symptoms with exertion before engaging in at-risk activities. The maximum heart rate (mHR) below is calculated as 220 minus the person's age.

Step 2

This step can start as early as twenty-four hours after the injury The concussed person resumes their typical physical activities (e.g., slow walking).

Step 3

The concussed person may start slow-to-medium paced walking and/or stationary bike workouts. They may gradually increase their aerobic exercise from light level (i.e., approximately 55 percent mHR, see chapter 3) to moderate level (i.e., 70 percent mHR, see chapter 3). They may also start light resistance training that does not result in more than mild and brief worsening of their symptoms.

Step 4

The concussed person can start sport-specific exercises and recreational activities (e.g., those involving running, training drills, and change of direction). In sport, such training activities should be done away from the team environment. For recreational activities, the concussed person should return to the activity outside of a group setting, where they have little control of what others will do. At this level, there should be no risk of head impact, and low risk of falling or being jarred. Prior to commencing this level, medical clearance is required if there is any risk of head impact.

For RTSR, steps 5–7 can only begin after there are no symptoms, no issues in cognition, and no other ongoing clinical findings related to the current concussion. These changes should not occur during and/or after activity. If all these conditions are not met, the concussed person should return to step 4 of RTCR.

<u>Step 5</u>

The concussed person can start noncontact activities that require higher intensity, coordination, and increased thinking (e.g., passing drills, multiplayer training). In sport, such training activities may be done in the team environment. For recreational activities, the concussed person may return to the activity in group settings.

<u>Step 6</u>

The concussed person can start activities that could involve full contact (e.g., normal team practices).

<u>Step 7</u>

The concussed person can return to sport and competitive play. Prior to embarking upon this final step, written readiness for full return to sport should be provided by a qHCP (directed by local laws and/or sporting regulations).

The general recommendations contained in this section are a very good foundation for how to return a child or youth to sport and recreation. But such provisions can be tricky to apply to different ages and situations. To this end, the following sections provide age-specific resources. If there is a contradiction between one guideline and another, I suggest you use the most up-to-date guideline. Naturally, as we learn more, our knowledge and practices need to evolve.

9.5 Returning Children to Activity

How quickly a child recovers depends on many, many factors, including the severity of their concussion, whether they experienced concussion-associated amnesia, the number of concussions they have had, the symptoms of ongoing fogginess and/or dizziness, the presence of migraines before or after the concussion, and a prior history of learning or behavioural problems.

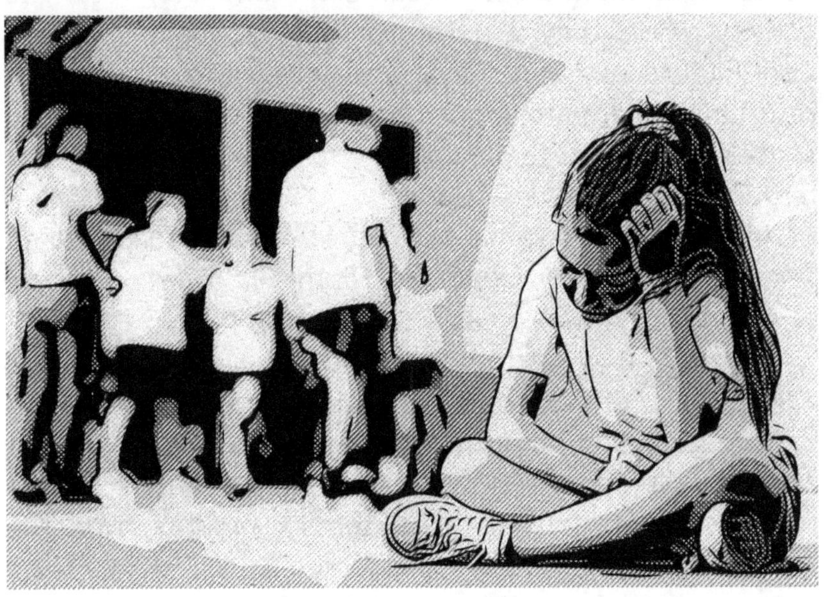

Using one-size-fits-all templates for returning children to activity does not work. As with return to school, it's essential that all involved parties (parents, educators, and clinicians) regularly check in with the student to find out how they are feeling and coping. Everyone, especially the child, needs to know that ignoring symptoms (i.e., the "suck it up" approach) is not a good idea. It can lead to prolonged issues and, in some cases, may completely stall recovery. There are some wonderful resources out there when it comes to returning children to sport. Rather than try to reinvent the wheel, I'm going to point out those that are most helpful.

McMaster's CanChild has well laid out and straightforward return-to-activity guidelines for children.[2] It outlines six distinct stages and includes when to move forward to the next stage, or when to move the child back to the previous level. For the first three stages, the CanChild guide recommends a child can simultaneously return to activity while they are returning to school. However, CanChild recommends that the latter three stages of returning children to sport wait until the child is fully (and *successfully*) back to school (see chapter 8). Other great features in this guide include: [2]

- An emphatic *no same day return to sport* following an event (also, *"If in doubt, sit them out"* rule).
- A series of time frames for how long to keep them out of sport and certain activities, based on specific criteria. For example, if the child has had two concussions in three months, then the child should not engage in sport and more risky recreational activities (e.g., rough-housing play) for six months from the time of the most recent incident.
- Examples of activities possible for each stage. In addition, a longer list of activities children can do at each stage is given elsewhere on the referenced site. This latter info is very useful for teachers and parents.
- Important red flags clinicians, teachers, and parents should look for.

9.6 Returning Youth and Adults to Sport

The Canchild recommendations can also be used for youth, particularly the younger ages. For older individuals, Parachute's Return to Sport Strategy [3] lays out six stages to return to sport. As with the CanChild Guide, it tells you as a minimum how long the individual is to stay in each stage, when to advance to the next stage, and what would indicate the person needs to drop back to an earlier stage. It recommends that anyone retuning to sport should never resume (especially contact practice) without a qualified physician's clearance. It gives resources for how to find such a knowledgeable doctor. At the above site, Parachute has some additional useful resources including [4]

- a series of "sport-specific return-to-sport guides," worked out in consultation with various sport organizations and governing bodies (e.g., Hockey Canada); and
- guides for parents, physicians, athletic directors, coaches, teachers, and other supervisors.

9.7 Baseline Testing

Baseline tests can be done for students (ten years and older) before they start a given season of team sport. In case of a concussion event, the baseline test results are then compared to their post-injury tests. Parachute, a national charity dedicated to injury prevention, has made the following statement about baseline testing: [5]

"Baseline testing using any tool or combination of tools is not required to provide post-injury care of those who sustain a suspected or diagnosed concussion, and mandatory preseason testing is not recommended. In general, current evidence does not support a significant added benefit of baseline testing of athletes . . . However, there may be unique athlete populations and sport environments where baseline testing may be considered."

Some of these exceptions include
- when a clinical neuropsychologist is involved in the testing and interpretation of the results; and

- for teams and sporting federations' multidisciplinary concussion programs with properly certified and experienced healthcare clinicians to administer and interpret these tests.

Finally, concussions come from many sources beyond team sports (e.g., falls, motor vehicle collisions, workplace injuries, etcetera) where concussions cannot be anticipated. Pretesting is therefore not practical for these.

References

1. Patricios J.S., et al. 2024. "Consensus Statement on Concussion in Sport: The 6th International Conference on Concussion in Sport–Amsterdam. October 2022." Br J Sports Med. 57, no. 11 (Jun), 695–711. https://doi.org/10.1136/bjsports-2023-106898
2. CanChild. 2024 "Brain Injury Resources." https://www.canchild.ca/en/diagnoses/brain-injury-concussion/brain-injury-resources/
3. Parachute. 2024. "Concussion Collection - Guides" https://www.parachute.ca/en/professional-resource/concussion-collection/?resources=guides
4. Parachute. 2024. "Concussion Collection - Concussion protocol resources for sport organizations." https://www.parachute.ca/en/professional-resource/concussion-collection/concussion-protocol-resources-for-sport-organizations/
5. Parachute. 2024. "Professional resources - Statement on Concussion Baseline Testing in Canada." https://www.parachute.ca/en/professional-resources/statement-on-concussion-baseline-testing-in-canada/

Appendices

Appendix A

See also https://www.paulgodlewski.com/concussion-exercise-tools-and-appendices/

Nine Things to Consider
(The Honey Approach)

- Individuals with concussion/PPCS will often look better on the outside long, long before they have fully recovered. How they feel will also fluctuate greatly. They will have their good days and their bad days, their good moments and not so good ones.

- Individuals with concussion/PPCS can easily get physically and/or mentally fatigued. They will need much more rest than they used to. Fatigue will make it hard for them to think, process, and organize. Pushing too hard may lead to flare-ups and setbacks.

- The time to recover will vary greatly. Sometimes it will be mere days or weeks. Other times it may take years. Try not to compare one person with concussion/PPCS with another. Recovery may also continue long after formal rehabilitation treatments have finished. They may or may not return to being exactly as they were. Expecting them to do so does not make it happen and puts a lot of stress on them for something that is often not in their control.

- Allow individuals with concussion/PPCS to find their own words and follow their own thoughts. Doing this will help them rebuild their memory and language skills. Not remembering something does not mean that they don't care about it.

- Occasions involving a lot of people in one place such as meetings, parties, religious services, and conferences can be very challenging for individuals with concussion/PPCS. They may resist social situations. This is because often such individuals are not able to filter and prioritize sounds and moving objects as well as before. If there is more than one person talking, they may not be able to follow the conversation. To have more time to process what has been said, they may request you give them a pause or break.

- Individuals with concussion/PPCS may sometimes appear rigid in the way they do things, but repetition is a strategy to getting better and will lead to more diverse ways of doing things later.

- Acting out can be an indication of their inability to deal with a specific situation or built-up frustration from a number of things. They may be experiencing a lot of symptoms at the time, be overloaded by stimuli, tired, confused, and/or frustrated. Multitasking is challenging for all of us, but particularly for the brain-injured. Patience is the best thing you can give them.

- Tasks that are normally automatic, which take little effort for the uninjured, will take them much, much more effort and time. If they seem sensitive or emotional, it may be a reflection of the much greater effort it takes to do things. Help them by encouraging them with all efforts. Try not to be too negative or critical. At that moment, they are likely doing the best they can.

- If a person with concussion/PPCS is having difficulty doing a task, doing it for them will not be constructive, and it will make them feel inadequate. If they appear stuck, asking what you can do to help may assist them in figuring it out. Sometimes it may work best if you leave them uninterrupted to work things out on their own, at their own pace.

Appendix B

See also https://www.paulgodlewski.com/concussion-exercise-tools-and-appendices/

Nine Things NOT to Say
(The Vinegar Approach)

Concussion is best thought of as a mild traumatic brain injury, not just a bump on the head. Brain injury is confusing to people who don't have one. It's natural to want to say something, to voice an opinion, or offer advice, even when we don't understand. And when you care for a loved one with a brain injury, it's easy to get burnt out and say things out of frustration. Here are nine things you should avoid saying to someone recovering from a concussion / Persistent Post-Concussive Symptoms.

- *You seem fine to me.* The invisible signs of a brain injury—memory and concentration problems, fatigue, insomnia, chronic pain, depression, or anxiety—are sometimes more difficult to live with than visible disabilities. Research shows that just having a scar on the head can help a person with a brain injury feel validated and better understood. Your loved one may look normal, but shrugging off the invisible signs of brain injury belittles the injured person.

- *Maybe you're just not trying hard enough (i.e., you're lazy).* Laziness is not the same as apathy (lack of interest, motivation, or emotion). Apathy is common after a brain injury. Apathy can often get in the way of rehabilitation and recovery, so it's important to recognize and treat it. Certain prescription drugs have been shown to reduce apathy. Setting very specific goals might also help. Beware of problems that mimic apathy. Depression, fatigue, and chronic pain are common after a brain injury and can look like (or be combined with) apathy. Side effects of some prescription drugs can also look like apathy. Try to discover the root of the problem so that you can help advocate for proper treatment.

- *You're such a grump!* Irritability is one of the most common signs of a brain injury. Irritability could be the direct result of the brain injury or a side effect of depression, anxiety, chronic pain, sleep disorders, or fatigue. Think of it as a biological grumpiness. It's hard to live with someone who is grumpy, moody, or angry all the time. Certain prescription drugs, supplements, changes in diet, or therapy that focuses on adjustment and coping skills can all help to reduce irritability.

- *How many times do I have to tell you?* It's frustrating to repeat yourself over and over, but almost everyone who has a brain injury will experience some memory problems. Instead of pointing out a deficit, try finding a solution. Make the task easier. Create a routine. Install a memo board in the kitchen. Also, remember that language isn't always verbal. "I've already told you this" comes through loud and clear just by facial expression.

- *Do you have any idea how much I do for you?* Your loved one probably knows how much you do and feels incredibly guilty about it. It's also possible that your loved one has no clue and may never understand. This can be due to problems with awareness, memory, or apathy—all of which can be a direct result of a brain injury. You do need to unload your burden on someone. Just let that someone be a good friend or a counsellor.

- *Your problem is all the medications you take.* Prescription drugs can cause all kinds of side effects such as sluggishness, insomnia, memory problems, mania, sexual dysfunction, or weight gain, just to name a few. Someone with a brain injury is especially sensitive to these effects. But, if you blame everything on the effects of drugs, two things could happen. One, you might be encouraging your loved one to stop taking an important drug prematurely. Two, you might be overlooking a genuine sign of brain injury. It's a good idea to regularly review prescription drugs with a doctor. Don't be afraid to ask about alternatives that might reduce side effects. At some point in recovery, it might very well be the right time to taper off a drug. But you won't know this without regular follow-up.

- *Let me do that for you.* Independence and control are two of the most important things lost after a brain injury. Yes, it may be easier to do things for your loved one. Yes, it may be less frustrating. But encouraging your loved one to do things on their own will promote self-esteem, confidence, and quality of living. It can also help the brain recover faster. Do make sure that the task isn't one that might put your loved one at genuine risk—such as driving too soon or managing medication when there are significant memory problems.

- *Try to think positively.* That's easier said than done for many people, and even harder for someone with a brain injury. Repetitive negative thinking is called rumination, and it can be common after a brain injury. Rumination is usually related to depression or anxiety, so treating those problems may help break the negative thinking cycle. Furthermore, if you tell someone to stop thinking a certain negative thought, that thought will just be pushed further toward the front of the mind (literally, to the prefrontal cortex). Instead, find a task that is especially enjoyable for your loved one. It will help to distract from negative thinking and release chemicals that promote more positive thoughts.

- *You're lucky to be alive.* This sounds like positive thinking, looking on the bright side of things. But be careful. A person with a brain injury is six times more likely to have suicidal thoughts than someone without a brain injury. Some may not feel very lucky to be alive. Instead of calling it "luck," talk about how strong, persistent, or heroic the person is for getting through their ordeal.

Appendix C

See also https://www.paulgodlewski.com/concussion-exercise-tools-and-appendices/

Symptom-Action Frameworks

Appropriate for Concussions (i.e., less than one month from injury)

Here are the four rules for you to follow during this period:

1. If you have a given symptom (a headache, say), be as active as you can, but try not to worsen the symptom. If it worsens, STOP, take five minutes rest (e.g., mini meditation), then switch to doing something different. If you were doing something mental (e.g., doing insurance paperwork—egad), switch to doing something physical (e.g., go for a walk—phew!).

2. If a new symptom appears, STOP and take five minutes' rest. Then switch to doing something different as above.

3. Pay attention to your symptoms the next day. If you wake up with stronger symptoms compared to the end of the day before, this means you have overdone it with the previous day's activities.

4. While doing specific exercises, your symptoms may increase. This is okay so long as the increase is

tolerable for you, and so long as your symptoms return to their pre-exercise level within about ten minutes. If not, you will need to decrease the difficulty, repetitions, duration, etcetera, so you don't break this fourth rule.

If you can't always follow these guidelines, don't worry, *you are not causing yourself harm*. You are not going to be perfect at this, but again, that's fine. These rules are recommended to speed up your recovery and are more important the newer your concussion is. The longer you have had your concussion (e.g., at one month on versus one week on), the less strictly you need to adhere to this guideline.

Appropriate for Persistent Post-Concussive Symptoms – PPCS (i.e., use this framework for one month or greater from the injury.)

Here are the four rules for you to follow during this period:

1. If you are experiencing annoying symptoms, your approach is to ignore them.

2. If you are experiencing aggravating symptoms, in other words, worse than just annoying but still tolerable, your approach is to try to put up with them.

3. If your symptoms become intolerable, you need to change your activities (in degree and/or duration), so that your symptoms are merely annoying or aggravating the next time around.

4. Avoidance is not the best policy at this stage. Moderating your activities is a better approach for PPCS.

Appendix D

See also https://www.paulgodlewski.com/concussion-exercise-tools-and-appendices/

Activity Versus Symptom Journal
(Plus or Minus Mood)

Three times a day, mark down your overall symptom level out of ten. You can circle if you are low in mood (LM) and/or anxious (A). This would be useful if you are consulting a psychological counsellor. In each time frame, note your activities, including the environment (e.g., noisy) and its duration.

	Morning	**Afternoon**	**Evening**
	Symptom / 10 **Mood** LM A	**Symptom** / 10 **Mood** LM A	**Symptom** / 10 **Mood** LM A
Day 1			
	Symptom / 10 **Mood** LM A	**Symptom** / 10 **Mood** LM A	**Symptom** / 10 **Mood** LM A
Day 2			

	Symptom / 10 **Mood** LM A	**Symptom** / 10 **Mood** LM A	**Symptom** / 10 **Mood** LM A
Day 3			
	Symptom / 10 **Mood** LM A	**Symptom** / 10 **Mood** LM A	**Symptom** / 10 **Mood** LM A
Day 4			
	Symptom / 10 **Mood** LM A	**Symptom** / 10 **Mood** LM A	**Symptom** / 10 **Mood** LM A
Day 5			
	Symptom / 10 **Mood** LM A	**Symptom** / 10 **Mood** LM A	**Symptom** / 10 **Mood** LM A
Day 6			
	Symptom / 10 **Mood** LM A	**Symptom** / 10 **Mood** LM A	**Symptom** / 10 **Mood** LM A
Day 7			

Appendix E

See also https://www.paulgodlewski.com/concussion-exercise-tools-and-appendices/

Week Ahead Planning Tool

Use to plan what you would optimally like to do. Start by filling in what you do regularly (e.g., get up, breakfast, etcetera). Then things you regularly have to do (e.g., children pickup, work, etcetera). Then add exercise and rest and relaxation times.

	MON	TUES	WED	THURS	FRID	SAT	SUN
06:00 - 06:30							
06:30 - 07:00							
07:00 - 07:30							
07:30 - 08:00							
08:00 - 08:30							
08:30 - 09:00							
09:00 - 09:30							
09:30 - 10:00							
10:00 - 10:30							
10:30 - 11:00							
11:00 - 11:30							
11:30 - 12:00							
12:00 - 12:30							
12:30 - 01:00							

01:00 - 01:30						
01:30 - 02:00						
02:00 - 02:30						
02:30 - 03:00						
03:00 - 03:30						
03:30 - 04:00						
04:00 - 04:30						
04:30 - 05:00						
05:00 - 05:30						
05:30 - 06:00						
06:00 - 06:30						
06:30 - 07:00						
07:00 - 07:30						
07:30 - 08:00						
08:00 - 08:30						
08:30 - 09:00						
09:00 - 09:30						
09:30 - 10:00						
10:00 - 10:30						
10:30 - 11:00						
11:00 - 11:30						
11:30 - 12:00						

Appendix F

See also https://www.paulgodlewski.com/concussion-exercise-tools-and-appendices/

The Hospital Anxiety and Depression Scale
(HADS)

For each question, draw a circle around the number of the answer that most closely resembles how you have been feeling in the past week. Don't take too long considering your replies. Your immediate response is best. Please note, the scoring is only valid if have drawn a circle for each of the questions.

Tick the box beside the reply that is closest to how you have been feeling in the past week.
Don't take too long over you replies: your immediate is best.

D	A		D	A	
		I feel tense or 'wound up':			I feel as if I am slowed down:
	3	Most of the time	3		Nearly all the time
	2	A lot of the time	2		Very often
	1	From time to time, occasionally	1		Sometimes
	0	Not at all	0		Not at all
		I still enjoy the things I used to enjoy:			I get a sort of frightened feeling like 'butterflies' in the stomach:
0		Definitely as much		0	Not at all
1		Not quite so much		1	Occasionally
2		Only a little		2	Quite Often
3		Hardly at all		3	Very Often
		I get a sort of frightened feeling as if something awful is about to happen:			I have lost interest in my appearance:
	3	Very definitely and quite badly	3		Definitely
	2	Yes, but not too badly	2		I don't take as much care as I should
	1	A little, but it doesn't worry me	1		I may not take quite as much care
	0	Not at all	0		I take just as much care as ever
		I can laugh and see the funny side of things:			I feel restless as I have to be on the move:
0		As much as I always could		3	Very much indeed
1		Not quite so much now		2	Quite a lot
2		Definitely not so much now		1	Not very much
3		Not at all		0	Not at all
		Worrying thoughts go through my mind:			I look forward with enjoyment to things:
	3	A great deal of the time	0		As much as I ever did
	2	A lot of the time	1		Rather less than I used to
	1	From time to time, but not too often	2		Definitely less than I used to
	0	Only occasionally	3		Hardly at all
		I feel cheerful:			I get sudden feelings of panic:
3		Not at all		3	Very often indeed
2		Not often		2	Quite often
1		Sometimes		1	Not very often
0		Most of the time		0	Not at all
		I can sit at ease and feel relaxed:			I can enjoy a good book or radio or TV program:
	0	Definitely	0		Often
	1	Usually	1		Sometimes
	2	Not Often	2		Not often
	3	Not at all	3		Very seldom

Please check you have answered all the questions

Scoring HADS

Add up all the numbers that you have circled in the columns marked with "D." This is tracking any possible issues you may be having with low mood. Now add up all the numbers you have circled in the columns marked with "A." This is tracking any possible issues you may be having with anxiety. *Hey! No changing your answers!*

If the total of your score for either "D" and/or "A" equal(s) zero to seven, you are considered to be at a normal mood level for both the low mood and anxiety poles.

If the total of your score for either "D" and/or "A" equal(s) eight to eleven, you may be having some issues with low mood and/or anxiety. In this case, I usually recommend that the patient self-monitor. If your poor mood and/or anxiety lingers for a while or worsens, I recommend you consult your GP and/or your psychological counsellor. *Be honest with yourself.*

If the total of your score for either "D" and/or "A" equal(s) twelve to twenty-one, you are definitely having issues with low mood and/or anxiety. In this case, consult your GP and/or your psychological counsellor. I recommend you take a copy of your HADS results to these consultations.

Appendix G

See also https://www.paulgodlewski.com/concussion-exercise-tools-and-appendices/

Letters and Numbers

Reference chapter 7 for the exercise instructions.

L 1 U K T	C 2 S O H
B P G 3 S	4 A U M T
A L D R 5	M S P 6 F
A M 7 E K	B D X R 8
9 N B C F	A E 10 G P
M P O E 11	12 C B K F
O T 13 P X	S V 14 A R
15 C M S F	T 16 R X B
A 17 K B M	F W T 18 E
X A L 19 E	20 A B Y T

Acknowledgments

I especially want to thank my wife, Beth Godlewski, and sister, Anne Godlewska. Both were invaluable in supporting and encouraging this endeavour, and in *patiently* reviewing and improving earlier drafts of this book.

All professionals rely on the generosity of experienced clinicians in teaching other less experienced members. This was no less the case for me in my early days of vestibular and concussion physiotherapy. Of particular importance to me was the mentoring of Bernard Tonks (PT) in vestibular rehabilitation therapy (VRT), and his encouragement to explore VRT's sister therapy, concussion physiotherapy. He also helped me by reviewing my chapter on dizziness. Shannon McGuire's (PT) postgraduate courses on concussion physiotherapy gave me a firm foundation and lots of practical material on which to build. I also want to acknowledge Carol Kennedy (PT), who showed me the importance of the neck in contributing to concussion issues.

Over the years, I have shared the care of my patients with many other professionals. Not only have my patients gained enormously from this multidisciplinary approach, I have learned a great deal collaborating with them. I routinely work with clinicians from a dozen professions. Members from all these groups generously agreed to review chapter(s) in their domains, including:

Bonnie Cai-Durant (PT), Patricia Bain and Melissa Cutler (Social work counsellors), Dr. Deborah Fisher (GP and headache management), Dr. Nathaniel Ibey (Sport MD), Dr. Alice Kam (Physiatrist), Elise Kopman (OT), Nurit Nader (SLP - cognitive assessment and treatment), Dr. Alex Osborn (Otolaryngologist), Dr. Angela Peddle (Neuro-optometrist), and Dr. Lesley Ruttan (Neuropsychologist).

Catherine Monahan greatly assisted me by giving me access to the latest medical and allied heath care literature. Michele Harms (PT and editor in chief of the journal *Physiotherapy*) helped to connect me to people in the publishing world. A big thank you to my editing and book formatting team at Polgarus Studios, particularly Marina Anderson who *patiently* answered my numerous questions about the publishing process.

Thanks to my colleagues at Trilogy Physiotherapy, West, Toronto: Jennifer Hunter, Diana Lupulovic, Brendan Pynenburg, and Jennifer Shtulberg for modelling my exercises. Finally, thanks to Jason Gallant, who kindly allowed me to do photography and video work at one of Trilogy's clinics.

About the Author

Paul Godlewski, PT (physiotherapist or physical therapist in the USA) is affectionately known locally as the *"Dizzio."* His expertise in vestibular and concussion physiotherapy is the very unforeseen highlight of two completely different career paths, spanning more than thirty-seven years.

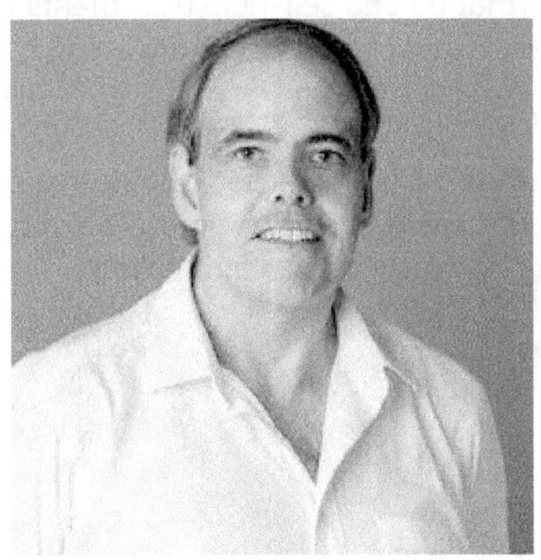

Educated in Canada, the USA, and the UK, he qualified in 1985 at McGill University in architecture. He practised as a commercial and residential architect for nine years. Interested in healing and physiology well before architecture, he came to realize he was also much more interested in people than the bricks and mortar of architectural practice. In his mid-thirties, he pulled up stakes and retrained as a physiotherapist, graduating with honours from the University of Toronto in 1998. Seeking greater skills and qualifications, he successfully completed VRT training at Emory University in Atlanta, Georgia, USA. With VRT's focus on neuroplastic recovery, it was a natural progression for him to work with concussions. In 2014, he successfully completed special postgraduate training in concussion physiotherapy.

He has been actively treating for twenty-five years. Given the high demand in Toronto, the focus of his private consultancy practice for the last ten years has been exclusively for concussion and vestibular clients. Nearing retirement, he now wants to pass on much-needed information and self-help treatments to the many concussed individuals who don't always have access to concussion-experienced clinicians.

Happily married to his wife Beth, they live and work in Toronto. Paul's main pastimes are gardening, travelling, an occasional game of tennis and skiing.

Index